Nursing expertise and advanced practice

Key Management Skills in Nursing

Other titles in this series

Dementia: Management for nurses and community care workers *by Dr Iain B McIntosh and Keith Woodall*
Management in the Acute Ward *by Jane Walton and Maggie Reeves*
Managing Continuing Education: a consumer's and provider's point of view *by Marilyn Williams*
Managing the Ethical Process in Research *by Marilyn Hammick*
Learning Skills, Studying Styles and Profiling *by Roswyn Brown and Barbara Hawksley*
Deep vein thrombosis: The silent killer *by Ricky Autar*
Managing Pressure Sore Prevention *by Carol Dealey*
Promoting Health: an issue for nursing *by Nicola Mackintosh*

Key Management Skills in Nursing

Edited by
Roswyn A Brown and George Castledine

Nursing expertise and advanced practice

by Jane E Conway

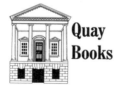

Quay
Books

Quay Books, Division of Mark Allen Publishing Limited
Jesses Farm, Snow Hill, Dinton, Nr Salisbury, Wilts, SP3 5HN

©Mark Allen Publishing Ltd, 1996
ISBN 1-85642-144 9

British Library Cataloguing-in-Publication Data
A catalogue record for this book is available from the British
Library

Printed in the UK by Beshara Press, Cheltenham

Contents

Acknowledgements

First, I would like to thank the expert nurses who participated in my study; without them this work would not have been possible. I would also like to thank Dawn Rafferty, Lyn Francis and Marilyn Williams for their comments and encouragement. Marilyn deserves a special mention for acting as a sounding board and for her continuous support. At a personal level thanks are due to my partner, David, for putting up with me throughout the whole composition process. Finally, I would like to thank my PhD supervisor, Chris Duke. His support, peppered with wry humour and cryptic comments, proved invaluable throughout my study.

Foreword

Mini doctor or maxi nurse? What will be the profile and responsibility of the expert nurse of the future? Jane Conway probes the 'hidden world of nursing' from within and poses questions crucially important for the future of the occupation and for the National Health Service. There are implications, not only for the preparation and support of nurses for an understanding of their role, but also for the preparation of doctors who need to be sensitised and oriented to work with their nurse colleagues. To jump prematurely to the conclusion of the book in respect of nurse development and support:

> *'if the "selective blindness of the oppressed" is to be overcome nurses need to be empowered so that they can cope with looking searchingly at themselves and their practice. Empowerment is much more than a popular cliché of the moment'* (Chapter 8, p119).

Dr Conway claims, with justice, to 'capture some of the specialness' of nursing, demonstrating the importance of, for instance, integrity and humanism, and exposing the reality of what expert nurses with a positive sense of their own self-worth can do.

This is a clarion call to those nurses who feel powerless and oppressed to change their working culture. As the book makes clear, given the traditional, often internalised, roles of (mostly female) nurses working with (traditionally male) doctors, this is by no means easy. Jane Conway's 'grounded' study of nurses, identified by their peers as expert, generated four 'bottom-up' practice-based models or 'types' of expert nurse. Her research followed them around the wards, watched them at work and listened to the way they perceived and reflected on what they were doing, why they did it, how they survived, the stratagems they employed, in particular, to cope with doctor colleagues. Listening to Jane Conway and following her research has been a fascinating, and at times a scary, experience. As a non-medic and one not overly fond of hospitals — a little too squeamish about operations and para-operational activities — I was left all too often distinctly and nervously uncomfortable. I became ever more appreciative that there were senior nurses around (who seem to me like the experienced NCOs of the health forces) to protect doctors — the young, and maybe sometimes the not-so-young, but perhaps just tired and too casual — from themselves, and their patients from them.

Some of the more alarming episodes uncovered during the research have been dropped from this published form of Dr Conway's work, to the partial relief of at least this reader. That does not detract from its interest or its utility. Real or reported crises in the Health Service and the bad, even fatal, experiences of some unlucky patients make this book's contents highly topical. In the changing Health Service of a none too wealthy or successful society, the development and support of expert nurses is an important, maybe literally vital, factor. If nurses are afraid to take responsibility, and need to resort at times to some of the stratagems revealed here to save their jobs and to try to do them properly, there is a real danger that cautious or 'defensive' practice will prove costly, even deadly, more often than we would care — or be allowed — to know. Dr Conway's study of nursing expertise and advanced practice contains important lessons and deserves to be widely read.

Chris Duke
University of Warwick
March 1996

Preface

This book seeks to challenge the accepted view that expertise can be somehow imported into practice. Rather, it argues that expertise development is much more complex, dependent on the expert's 'world view'. The aim of this work is to highlight the influence of socialisation and organisational culture on the use and development of nursing knowledge.

The extension of nursing roles has been the focus for considerable media attention recently. This work explores the world of advanced practice and ascertains how boundaries between medicine and nursing are re-adjusting.

Current concerns within the NHS about quality assurance and value for money mean that nursing needs to identify the 'uniqueness' of the nursing role. This account identifies, through the use of examples, what is expert about nursing practice. The aim is to establish that quality is linked to the reflective ability of the expert nurse and this, in turn, is linked to their 'world view'.

Introduction

A silk purse or a sow's ear — what is special about nursing practice?

In the past, nursing practice was taken for granted. Training involved the acquisition of knowledge from outside the practice setting, often from other disciplines, particularly medicine. Nursing was what nurses were trained to do. Such perceptions demonstrated a singular lack of curiosity in relation to practice and no longer have a place in nursing today.

This has occurred largely because nursing has undergone major change during the last ten years as a result of two main influences. First, reorganisation of the National Health Service (NHS) (Griffiths, 1983) in line with market forces has been influential. This requires nurses to articulate the value of nursing practice. Secondly, the drive for professionalisation and academic recognition within nursing itself (UKCC, 1986; ENB 1991; UKCC, 1994) has promoted substantial change often focused directly on practice.

The introduction of market forces, with nursing care seen in cost effective terms, requires nurses to articulate the value of nursing in a way that was previously unimaginable (DHSS, 1989). The challenge is to present the complexity of factors which make up nursing into a form that can be quantified.

This is no mean task. The danger is that in attempting to reduce nursing to descriptive terms and competences, much of the richness that makes up practice will be lost.

The reduction in junior doctors' hours (Greenhalgh, 1994) has also had a major influence on the nature of nursing practice. In many areas nurses are bridging the gap produced by this reduction. Nurses are being encouraged to extend the scope of their practice and to make their own decisions as to their competence to carry out tasks previously within the province of doctors. New qualifications related to practice are springing up for nurses. In addition, learning is now seen as a life-long process and the attainment of Advanced Practice is seen as a goal for many.

How aware the general public is about such changes is far from clear. If the media reflect public opinion, then some reports of nurses extending and expanding their roles have been received with incredulity. 'Nurse removes appendix' and other such headlines demonstrate that public expectations of the nurse's role may be falling behind practice initiatives.

Against this backdrop this work has arisen. It explores the nature of expert practical nursing knowledge. Factors which influence the development of expertise in the work place are considered. In addition the influence of nurses' 'world views' on practical knowledge are explored. It has never before been so important for nurses to reflect on these factors which are influencing their development, both negatively and positively. It is only with such knowledge that they can chart their own voyage through the sea of change in which they find themselves today. This work attempts to provide some guidance on that journey. Light is shed on some of the rocky areas and experienced travellers provide stories of their journeys to assist others.

References

Department of Health and Social Security (1989) *Working for Patients*. HMSO, London

English National Board (1991b) *Framework for Continuing Professional Education for Nurses, Midwives and Health Visitors: Guide to Implementation* ENB, London

Greenhalgh Co Ltd, Management Consultants (1994) *The Interface Between Junior Doctors and Nurses: A Research Study for the Department of Health*, Vol 1: report. DoH, London

Griffiths ER (1983) *NHS Management Inquire*: (letter to the Secretary of State). The Team, London

United Kingdom Central Council for Nursing, Midwifery and Health Visiting (1986) *Project 2000: A New Preparation for Practice*. UKCC, London

United Kingdom Central Council for Nursing, Midwifery and Health Visiting (1994) *PREP Recommendations April*. UKCC, London

Chapter 1

Defining terms: expert, specialist and advanced nurse — where are they going and what do they mean?

The literature related to developing nursing practice is scattered with many different names and titles. Terms such as specialist, advanced practitioner and expert are often used interchangeably (Sutton and Smith, 1995). Similarly, titles such as clinical nurse specialist, nurse practitioner and lecturer practitioner indicate that the holder possesses some type of advanced knowledge and/or skills. While some of these roles have been operational for the past hundred years (Chickadonz and Perry, 1985) confusion exists as to their similarities and differences. This is not just a problem in the UK; contributions from the USA (Steele and Fenton, 1988), Canada (Patterson and Haddad, 1992) and Australia (Sutton and Smith, 1995) share similar concerns.

The recent introduction by the United Kingdom Central Council (UKCC) (1994) of Specialist and Advanced Practice could have been expected to clarify the issues in the UK. However, parallel initiatives such as the development of the Higher Award (ENB, 1991), the introduction of Nurse Practitioners and Advanced Practice courses further complicate rather than clarify the issues.

Through examination of the literature and discussion with those studying for advanced practice and curriculum enquiry, the following points have emerged.

Expert practice and experience

Benner's work has been highly influential in terms of describing expertise. She presents nursing expertise as context specific and avoids describing characteristics of experts. Rather she presents scenarios within which expertise is demonstrated (Benner, 1984). Perceptual ability, pattern recognition and intuitive abilities are linked to expertise in nursing. Jasper (1994: 771) is not so reticent and defines expertise as:

'1.   *Possession of a specialised body of knowledge or skill.*

2.   *Extensive experience on that field of practice.*

3.   *Highly developed levels of pattern recognition.*

4.   *Recognition by others.'*

Both criteria encompass the notion of experience being central to the development of expertise. This perspective is supported by Schon's (1983; 1987) work on 'knowing-in-action' and 'reflection-in-action' where the professional, over time, encounters similar situations and develops a repertoire of knowledge about what is 'normal' in such a situation. This enables him/her to quickly detect when something occurs which is not normal and s/he is able to respond to this by synthesising theoretical and experiential knowledge. Schon calls this 'reflection-in-action'. In contrast to Benner (1984) and Jasper (1994) Conway found that expertise was not definitive. Rather, it developed differently depending upon the prevailing conditions. She saw this as an evolutionary process dependent on the 'world view' held by the expert nurse. This is explored more fully in Chapter 2.

Specialist practice

As the name originally denoted, specialist practice implies that the practitioner has developed specialist knowledge related to an area in which s/he works. Since the 1960s with the growth of high technology units, there has been increasing specialisation. Nurses have specialised in coronary care, intensive care, renal nursing, neurology and special care baby units to name but a few. The English National Board developed courses to prepare nurses within specialities. These were largely concerned with imparting speciality specific knowledge.

Recent recommendations about the role of the specialist nurse (Wallace and Gough, 1995) demonstrate a reappraisal of this role and reflect thinking expressed by Chickadonz and Perry in the USA way back in 1985. Not only was knowledge about a speciality seen as significant, but management and research abilities were also presented as integral to the role. Wallace and Gough (1995) outline the proposed eclectic nature of specialist practice:

> *'The specialist practitioner will be the team leader, and facilitator of innovative and creative practice in response to patient/client need, and will monitor and improve standards of care through supervision of practice, the provision of skilled professional leadership and the development of practice through clinical audit,*

research, teaching and the support of professional colleagues.'

Specialist practice in this description has strong professional and management components and is about much more than the speciality in which the nurse is working. Education and research are also presented as integral to the role. Such practitioners need to be able to:

'...exercise higher levels of judgement and discretion in clinical care ...demonstrate higher levels of clinical decision-making and ...be able to monitor and improve standards of care through supervision of practice, clinical nursing audit, developing and leading practice, contributing to research, teaching and supporting professional colleagues' (UKCC, 1994).

To facilitate such developments, degree level programmes which concentrate on the four broad areas of clinical nursing practice, care and programme management, clinical practice development and clinical practice leadership (UKCC, 1994) have been proposed and are in the process of development. This scheme provides a framework within which a more holistic approach to specialist practice is possible.

While the UKCC has been developing the nursing role in terms of specialist practice, wider social forces have promoted the emergence of nurse practitioners. It is argued that:

'The introduction of the term "nurse practitioner" with its vague definition, has allowed doctors to develop new roles for nurses. The rationale used most frequently ...has emphasised the... [need] to reduce junior doctors' hours and to save money' (Castledine, 1995).

Indeed, the introduction of *Scope of Professional Practice* (UKCC, 1992) and the reduction in junior doctors' hours (Greenhalgh, 1994) has opened the way for nurses to extend their roles dramatically. Such extension is now taking place throughout the country and nurses view this in different ways. Discussion with colleagues revealed that some see this development as an excellent way to provide a more holistic focus to care. Others see these tasks as being imposed on them and feel unprepared to take them on. They do so only because they feel that they have no choice.

Castledine (1995) asks 'Will the nurse practitioner be a mini doctor or a maxi nurse?' This is a crucial question and one which requires serious consideration by the profession. It also has relevance to the way the concept of advanced practice is being developed at the moment. This will be discussed further in the following section.

Advanced practice

> *'Advanced practice is concerned with adjusting the boundaries for the development of future practice, pioneering and developing new roles responsive to changing needs and with advancing clinical practice, research and education to enrich professional practice as a whole'* (UKCC, 1994).

The reader might be forgiven for asking 'what exactly does the above statement mean?' As if anticipating confusion, the UKCC goes on to explain that:

> *'Advanced practice will also make a contribution to health policy and management and in the determination of health need. This is not an additional layer of practice to be superimposed on specialist practice. It is rather, a description of an important sphere of professional practice, which is concerned with continuing development of the professions in the interests of clients, patients and the health services'* (UKCC, 1994).

Study at Masters' degree level is proposed for this role, but there will not be a specific qualification recorded on the register.

Exactly where advanced practice sits in relation to specialist practice is not clear. From the definitions it would seem possible to be both a specialist practitioner and an advanced practitioner at the same time. The only clear demarcation between the two seems to be that of the level of the degree undertaken, ie. first degree level for a specialist practitioner and Masters degree level for an advanced practitioner.

There are, however, drawbacks to such academic classifications: professional practice and academic levels do not necessarily correlate. In a study of expert practice Conway (1995) found that four types of expertise developed and these were not only linked to education and experience, but to other factors as well.There is a danger that because of the UKCC (1994) linkage, this will be overlooked and professional practice and academic levels will be assumed to be one and the same thing.

Nature of advanced practice

Two models are clearly emerging in terms of advanced practice and tensions arise between them. The medical model is demonstrably significant in some advanced practice curricula. Emphasis here is placed on nurses taking on doctors' tasks safely. What can easily be lost with such initiatives, however, is a nursing focus to care. Other advanced practice curricula demonstrate a nursing-focused approach to developing care based on a reflective paradigm. Such initiatives have their roots in nursing development units such as Burford (Johns, 1991) and in the work of Benner (1984) and Schon (1983; 1987). There are few links between these two models. They mirror the question posed by Castledine, see page 4:'Do nurses want to be mini doctors or maxi nurses?' The divisions go deep. The value of the nursing role, the nature of the nurse-patient relationship, therapeutic use of self, the importance of advocacy are all implicit in nursing models of advance practice. In contrast, an imposed medical model fosters the notion of nurses being assistants to medics and of medical knowledge being more important than the more qualitative aspects of nursing knowledge.

There are similarities, however, between the medical model of advanced practice and the Technologists described in chapter 2. There are also strong links between the Humanistic Existentialists, the UKCC (1994) definition of advanced practice and nursing-focused advanced practice programmes such as that run at the University of Central England.

We need to be very clear as to the type of nursing that we are trying to develop and to pursue this, rather than be overtaken by short-term opportunism. While such initiatives may enable us to bask in reflected medical glory, they will do little more than this. We need to determine the agenda and ensure that any nurse extension is integrated within a nursing approach to care.

References

Benner P (1984) *From Novice to Expert: Excellence and Power in Clinical Practice*. Addison-Wesley, California

Conway JE (1995) *Expert Nursing Knowledge as an Evolutionary Process*. Unpublished PhD Thesis, University of Warwick

Castledine G (1995) Will the nurse practitioner be a mini doctor or a maxi nurse? *Br J Nurs* 4(16): 938–9

Chickadonz GH, Perry AM (1985) Clinical Specialisation versus Generalisation: Perspectives for the Future. In: McCloskey JC, ed, *Current Issues in Nursing*. Blackwell Scientific, London

English National Board (1991) *Framework for Continuing Professional Education for Nurses, Midwives and Health Visitors.* ENB, London

Greenhalgh Co Ltd, Management Consultants (1994) *The Interface Between Junior Doctors and Nurses: A Research Study for the Department of Health,* Vol 1: Report. DOH, London

Jasper MA (1994) Expert: a discussion of the implications of the concept as used in nursing. *J Adv Nurs* **20**: 769–76

Johns C (1991) The Burford Nursing Development Unit holistic model of nursing practice. *J Adv Pract* **16**: 1090–8

Schon DA (1983) *The Reflective Practitioner: How Professionals Think in Action.* Basic Books Inc, New York

Schon DA (1987) *Educating the Reflective Practitioner.* Jossey-Bass, London

Steele S, Fenton MV (1988) Expert practice of clinical nurse specialists. *Clin Nurse Spec* **2**(1): 45–51

Sutton F, Smith C (1995) Advanced nursing practice: new ideas and new perspectives. *J Adv Nurs* **21**: 1037–43

Patterson C, Haddad B (1992) The advanced nurse practitioner: common attributes. *Can J Nurs Admin* Nov/Dec: 18–21

United Kingdom Central Council for Nursing, Midwifery and Health Visiting (1992) *The Scope of Professional Practice.* UKCC, London

United Kingdom Central Council for Nursing, Midwifery and Health Visiting (1994) *The Future of Professional Practice — The Council's Standards for Education and Practice Following Registration.* UKCC, London

Wallace M, Gough P (1995) The UKCC's criteria for specialist and advanced nursing practice. *Br J Nurs* **4**(16): 939–44

Chapter 2

Evolution of the species — expert nurse

This chapter describes a study carried out by Conway which examines the knowledge expert nurses use in practice. The study has been chosen to illustrate the evolution of the expert nurse because its findings highlight important points about advancing practice and developing expertise. A brief overview of the methodology is given, and the strategies and approaches used to ensure rigour are discussed. The findings are then considered.

Background to the Study

One of the first tasks of this study was to collect a group of experts. We all have our own beliefs and agendas when it comes to defining expertise, so the concern was to ensure that the experts were not chosen by one, perhaps biased, group. Therefore, rather than defining expertise herself, Conway asked managers, nurses and link educationalists to define what they meant by a practical nursing expert and to name such an expert from their area. A total of 913 respondents were consulted and 257 nominations were returned.

Through cross-referencing 40 expert nurses were named and of these 35 participated in the study.

The experts were selected from two authorities, one in the Midlands and the other in the South of England. These authorities were chosen because one was known to the author and was convenient for investigation. The other was a deviant sample (Patton, 1987:52) chosen because of its reputation for excellence in practice.

Literature review

Although this was an inductive study, an extensive review of the literature was carried out to inform the methodology and establish the current thinking in terms of practical nursing knowledge. This involved the examination of literature related to a number of disciplines and occupational groups, for example psychology (Chi *et al* 1981; 1982), sociology (Cervero, 1988), philosophy, management (Klemp and McClelland, 1986), teaching (Eraut, 1985; Shulman, 1986; Sockett, 1987; Nolan and Huber, 1989) and nursing (Carper, 1978; Benner, 1984; Howie, 1988; Brykczynski, 1989; Nehring, 1990; Davis *et al*, 1990; Fitzpatrick *et al*, 1992; Meerabeau, 1992; Davies, 1993; Shay and Stallings, 1993; Butterworth *et al*, 1993). A number of topic areas were investigated including types and sources of practical knowledge, reflection, accreditation, role models, competencies, expertise and intuition.

A number of issues arose from the literature. First, practical knowledge was defined in many ways and there was little consistency between definitions. The process of reflection was seen as central to learning from practice and to developing knowledge in the practice setting. Difficulties arose because the term 'reflection' was also presented in many ways and meant different things to different writers. Some associated it with pondering on events while others saw it as much more than this, eg. linked to action and as an attribute of professional practice (Schon, 1987). Values

(Raya, 1990), artistry (Schon, 1987) and intuition (Benner, 1984; Rew and Barrow, 1987; Rew, 1989) were all linked to the concept of expertise.

Methodology

There are many inconsistencies and ambiguities in the literature on qualitative methodologies, thus making informed choice a process fraught with difficulty. Terms such as 'phenomenology' and 'hermeneutics' have both generic and specific meanings and authors present these in different ways (Benner, 1984; Baker *et al*, 1992; Beck, 1994; Titchen and McIntyre, 1993). There are also sub-classifications within the terminology (Allen and Jensen, 1990).

Consequently operationalisation of a particular methodology within phenomenology is problematic. Also, there is little direction available as to if and how methodologies can be combined. Further, while examples of methods usage are provided as a means of ensuring rigour, this leads to confusion when the specific methodology used is not fully located within the total field of phenomenology (Titchen and McIntyre, 1993). As a result of these constraints, the development and use of an eclectic methodology was very much a learning process for the researcher. Ethnography, hermeneutic phenomenology and grounded theory were used.

Koch recently expressed methodological concerns regarding the philosophical underpinnings of a number of nursing studies. She suggested that to date nursing has largely defined phenomenological research:

> '... *by its techniques and procedures alone (Lynch-Sauer 1985; Hasse, 1987; Banonis, 1989; Hilton, 1988; Santopinto, 1988). This is possibly a characteristic of an emerging discipline, which concerns itself with "method" rather than exploring the theoretical or philosophical underpinnings*'(Koch, 1995).

This emphasis on method was an element in this study for pragmatic reasons. As the study was to inform curriculum and educational activities (Conway 1995), it was necessary to obtain both etic and emic perceptions of expert nursing knowledge. The insider's view was obtained through the use of critical incidents and interviews within the framework of phenomenology while the outsider's view was obtained through participant observation as used in ethnography.

However, such combining of methodologies has been criticised and described as method slurring:

'To ensure rigour ... qualitative data collection procedures should be explicit and consistent with the underlying assumptions of the specific approach selected' (Baker *et al, 1992).*

While such criticisms have justification, this has to be balanced against the needs of 'real world' environments that require some form of 'objectivity' within the research design. Consequently, pragmatic approaches to methodology are necessary at times. Although this requires compromise for those using hermeneutic methodology, the success of studies such as Benner's (1984) *Novice to Expert*, which combined phenomenology and grounded theory prove the benefits of such approaches. Benner's approach has been described as hermeneutics practised outside of the hermeneutic circle (Koch, 1995). By combining methodologies, it went beyond phenomenological description to theory generation.

The notion of the researcher as a bricoleur captures the essence of this pragmatic approach to methodology:

'The multiple methodologies of qualitative research may be viewed as a bricolage, and the researcher as a bricoleur' (Denzin and Lincoln, 1994).

This is clarified as the researcher being a 'jack-of-all-trades', a professional 'do-it yourself person' (Levi-Strauss 1966, cited by Denzin and Lincoln, 1994). The ability to self-build is an important one to nursing which has not as yet developed its own research methodology but instead uses methods 'borrowed' from other disciplines. Often, these only partly fit the requirements of nursing investigations.

A total of 165 hours was spent in observation visits, workshops and interviews. In addition, 80 hours of verbatim tape-recordings were transcribed. In retrospect it is clear that the use of observation, combined with critical incident technique and interviews, enabled inconsistencies between what expert nurses believed they did and what they actually did, to be recognised. These would not have been identified by the use of hermeneutic phenomenology alone.

Ensuring rigour

There is a common misconception in some circles that qualitative studies are somehow less rigorous than quantitative work. This is not necessarily the case. To ensure reliability and validity in this work, a number of strategies were employed based on the recommendations of Guba and Lincoln (1981), prominent theorists in this area. These included the use of purposive sampling, grounded theory and contextual interpretation (Lincoln and Guba, 1985). Repeated observation and prolonged engagement (Speizman cited by Guba and Lincoln, 1981: 105) were also used. Personal validity and validity and supervision (Reason and Rowan, 1981: 147) were considered. Data triangulation was used to ensure face validity (Munhall and Oiler, 1986: 159). In addition, verification with source, fittingness, auditability and confirmability (Guba and Lincoln, 1981: 126) were used to provide a rigorous base to this work.

Evolution of expertise

Expertise is not definitive. Rather, it develops in a number of ways in response to the 'world view' held by the expert. This acts as a process of selection in an evolutionary manner. In some areas knowledge use and development was at survival level only. In others, however, where the 'world view' was more favourable, expertise of a more sophisticated nature developed.

World view

The 'world views' of practitioners were developed from the orientation of the expert in terms of:

1. The philosophy and values held by the expert nurse and the organisation.

2. The type of model that shaped care delivery; that is either a medical or a nursing focus.

3. The goals of the expert nurse and the organisation.

4. The reflective ability of the expert nurse.

5. The level and type of education both professional and academic of the expert nurse.

6. The resources available to the expert nurse.

7. The relationship that expert nurses held with significant others such as doctors and managers.

8. The amount of authority which the expert nurse was able to exercise.

Four distinct types of expert emerged from the data and have been named Technologists, Traditionalists, Specialists and Humanistic Existentialists as these names encapsulate the characteristics exhibited.

Technologists

A wide range of knowledge was demonstrated by Technologists and included anticipatory knowledge, diagnosis knowledge, 'know-how' knowledge and monitoring knowledge both of junior doctors and patients' conditions. An expert anaesthetic nurse described this anticipatory knowledge:

> 'When you have enough knowledge, you will pick up the warning signs about a patient as quickly and sometimes quicker than a junior anaesthetist. Your hand will be on what he needs as he says it and it will be in his hand.'

Teaching by these experts was mainly didactic: images were used, as was in-depth questioning and a translator function was demonstrated. Issues arose in relation to the authority that expert nurses had vis-à-vis doctors.

Traditionalists

Expertise was demonstrated in terms of 'survival'. These experts were preoccupied with 'getting the work done' and managing care with scarce resources. In carrying out a task, care had a medical focus and the experts operated as overseers and doctors' assistants. Management and doctors were perceived as all powerful. They did not value their own practice and saw themselves as powerless in terms of influence. They saw education as an optional extra and not as central to practice development. Value was attached to 'doing' and not to 'reflecting'. They showed that 'papering-over-the-cracks' was what nursing was about and this others also learned to do. The dispossessed dispossessed others.

Specialists

These experts were prescribing treatment regimes, recommending medication and extending their roles. One expert, for example, was inserting her own central venous lines. There were subdivisions within this group that reflected the Traditionalists, Technologists and Humanistic Existentialists. They had developed knowledge in terms of assessment, diagnosing, quality of life and transformative ability. Doctor-nurse relationships varied. An expert total parenteral nutrition nurse discussed some of the influencing factors in terms of extending her role:

> 'One of the first things was to make it an economic gesture really, you see in the past it used to cost something like £400 to put in a line in theatre. I know the business manager has got it wrong because she is only charging for my services. She is charging £23 per patient which is absolutely ludicrous but we will get it right. By the way we are doing it we are keeping patients out of theatre; we are reducing their anaesthetic risk because there is none, and they are able to have their lines put in on the ward that they are familiar with, with nurses around them that they know and they feel very much more confident about the whole thing, which has to be good for them.'

Humanistic existentialists

These were very dynamic and had a strong nursing focus to care. Patients were truly viewed holistically and a humanistic philosophy was used in practice. These experts were passionate about nursing practice. A devolved hierarchy using primary nursing was operational. Humanistic Existentialist experts were risk takers. They had supportive management, good resources and were educationally well developed. They exerted considerable power and influence, and saw themselves as creating the culture in their areas.

Self-awareness and reflective abilities typified this group. They were also very aware of the influence which they had on other nurses.

Philosophies

Many of the experts (Traditionalists, some Technologists and Specialists) espoused philosophies which differed from their philosophies-in-use, ie. they said that they believed in one thing but went on to do another. They also perceived management as saying one thing and meaning another. For example, management's perceptions of quality translated into scant support and scarce resources. However, the experts were unable to see the difference between their own espoused beliefs — that they gave individualised care — and their own philosophies-in-action. These often demonstrated the opposite view, and showed that many of them valued care which was pragmatic, controlling, talk-allocated, medically-dominated and largely based on ritual and routine. The goals of the experts reflected the model of care from which they operated. Some were concerned with 'papering-over the cracks' and coping with scarce resources while others gave sophisticated patient-centred holistic care.

Reflective ability

All of the experts believed that they were reflective — this was not the case. There was scant evidence of this ability in the Traditionalists. There was some evidence in the Technologists and Specialists but it was mainly of a problem-solving nature. Reflective ability was the hallmark of the Humanistic Existentialists.

The lack of insight shown by many of the experts was the antithesis of critical reflectivity and denoted a type of blindness in relation to their beliefs and practice. Conway calls this 'the selective blindness of the oppressed'. Their belief that they were reflective enabled them to continue practising as they did. It was a means of reconciling and avoiding cognitive dissonance which arose from the unrealistic expectations placed on them.

The wider issues of emancipation, justice and political factors (Goodman, 1984) had relevance and coherence only to those practitioners who were sufficiently empowered to be able to question themselves and others. Variations in reflective ability characterised a transition from a training-based to a professional model of expertise. Those with minimal reflective abilities gave care which was limited in focus and illness-orientated. In contrast, reflective practitioners gave responsive care, full of warmth, based on the needs of the individual.

Points for consideration

What is the significance of this study for nursing and nursing education? Some might argue that not all of these groups reflect nursing expertise. However, each of the experts was nominated as such by an educationalist, a practitioner from their own area and a manager. The consensus, therefore, is that they are expert. Much as beauty is perceived in the eye of the beholder, so too is expertise. While choosing an expert is an entirely subjective process, it is likely to reflect the norms and values held within an organisation. As H G Wells so aptly put it 'in the country of the blind the one-eyed man is king'. Expertise development, therefore, is about not only ability and motivation at an individual level, but also the socialisation process within the care setting.

If we truly wish to develop expertise which is based on humanism and is holistic in nature, then a number of factors require attention. Nurses need to experience such philosophies in their own working lives: humanism has to be part of their reality and not just something which they read about in a book or discuss in the classroom. The complexity of knowledge use and development in the practice setting needs to be recognised: while education is necessary in this process, it is not sufficient on its own. The entirety of the 'world view' has to be considered. Empowerment needs to be central to developing humanistic and holistic expertise. Indeed, the whole learning milieu at care level has to support it. Management have a responsibility here. They need to be aware of the implications of scarce resources and lack of support on knowledge use and development. Also, if educational input is to be successful, it must be supported at ward level by management strategies and procedures: nurses need to feel supported and valued, not subjugated.

Innovative curriculum changes are also required. Emphasis needs to move from simple importation of knowledge to facilitating empowerment of practitioners. Practitioners need to be able to see their situation with their own eyes. However, such enlightenment carries a price and educationalists and professional bodies need to ensure that, with new consciousness, practitioners are given support. Curriculum also needs to be responsive to the present economic and political climate. It is little wonder that many nurses feel powerless to influence their situation when cultural and political dimensions of nursing are so rarely recognised or seen as influential. Both implicitly and explicitly curriculum needs to be critically reflective. This will demand much from educationalists.

Without such revision, unquestioning acceptance of the *status quo* will continue. Challenging and questioning has to be part of the reality in which nurses learn and work. This can only be accomplished by nurses gaining awareness of their own collective power and influence. Such enlightenment is necessary to enable nurses to become political animals so that they can survive in the present economic and political climate without sacrificing their professional or personal integrity. If we wish to foster the development of the species 'expert nurse' we need to ensure that we provide the necessary conditions for it to grow and flourish. The professional genus of the species does not breed well in impoverished environments. Indeed, this may result in its extinction. Other forms of the species are developing but they do not have the distinctive attributes of the professional genus of the species.

References

Allen MN, Jensen L (1990) Hermeneutical inquiry meaning and scope. *W J Nurs Res* **12(2)**: 242–53

Baker C, Wuest J, Noerager Stern P (1992) Method slurring: the grounded theory/phenomenology example. *J Adv Nurs* **17**: 1355

Beck CT (1994) Phenomenology: its use in nursing research. *Intl J Nurs Stud* **6**: 499–510

Benner P (1984) *From Novice to Expert: Excellence and Power in Clinical Practice*. Addison-Wesley, California

Butterworth CA (1993) *A Delphi Survey of Optimum Practice in Nursing, Midwifery and Health Visiting*. Executive Report, University of Manchester

Brykczynski KA (1989) An interpretive study describing the clinical judgement of nurse practitioners. *Schol Inq Nurs Pract Intl J* **3**(2): 75–103

Carper BA (1978) Fundamental patterns of knowing in nursing. *Adv Nurs Sci* **1**(1): 13–23

Cervero RM (1988) *Effective Continuing Education for Professionals*. Jossey-Bass, London

Chi MTH, Glaser R, Rees E (1981) Expertise in Problem Solving. In: *Advances in the Psychology of Human Intelligence*, vol 1. Erlbaum, Hills-dale, NJ

Davies E (1993) Clinical role modelling: uncovering hidden knowledge. *J Adv Nurs* **18**: 627–36

Davis AJ, Hershberger A, Ghan LC, Lin JY (1990) The good nurse: descriptions from the People's Republic of China. *J Adv Nurs* **15**: 829–34

Denzin NK, Lincoln YS eds (1994) *Handbook of Qualitative Research*. Sage Publications, London

Errant M (1985) Knowledge creation and knowledge use in professional contexts. *Stud H Educ* **10 (2)**: 117–33

Fitzpatrick J, While AE, Roberts JD (1992) The role of the nurse in high-quality patient care: a review of the literature. *J Adv Nurs* **17**: 1210–9

Glaser B, Strauss AL (1967) *The Discovery of Grounded Theory*. Aldine Publishing Co, Chicago

Goodman J (1984) Reflection and teacher education: a case study and theoretical analysis. *Interchange* **15**: 9–25

Guba EG, Lincoln YS (1981) *Effective Evaluation*. Jossey-Bass, London

Howie J (1988) The effective clinical teacher: a role model. *Aus J Adv Nurs* **5**(2): 23–6

Klemp GO, McClelland DC (1986) What Characterises Intelligent Functioning among Senior Managers. In: Sternberg RJ, Wagner RK eds, *Practical Intelligence — Nature and Origins of Competence in the Everyday World*, Part 1–3. Cambridge University Press, Cambridge: 31–50

Koch T (1995) Interpretive approaches in nursing research: the influence of Husserl and Heidegger. *J Adv Nurs* **21**: 827–36

Lincoln YS, Guba EG (1985) *Naturalistic Inquiry*. Sage Publications, London

Meerabeau L (1992) Tacit nursing knowledge: an untapped resource or a methodological headache? *J Adv Nurs* **17**: 108–12

Munhall PI, Oiler CJ (1986) *Nursing Research: A Qualitative Perspective*. Appleton-Century-Crofts, Connecticut

Nehring V (1990) Nursing clinical teacher effectiveness inventory: a replication study of the characteristics of 'best' and 'worst' clinical teachers as perceived by nursing faculty and students. *J Adv Nurs* **15**: 934–40

Nolan JF, Huber T (1989) Nurturing the reflective practitioner through instruction supervision: a review of the literature. *J Curriculum Supervision* 4(2): 126–45

Patton MQ (1987) *How to Use Qualitative Methods in Evaluation*. Sage Publications Inc, London

Raya A (1990) Can knowledge be promoted and values ignored? Implications for nursing education. *J Adv Pract* **15**: 505–9

Reason P, Rowan J eds (1981) *Human Enquiry: A Source Book of New Paradigm Research*. John Wiley & Sons, Chichester

Rew L (1989) Intuition: nursing knowledge and the spiritual dimension of persons. *Hol Nurs Pract* **3 (3)**: 56–68

Rew L, Barrow EM (1987) Intuition: a neglected hallmark of nursing knowledge. *Adv Nurs Sci* **10(1)**: 49–62

Schon DA (1987) *Educating the Reflective Practitioner*. Jossey-Bass, London

Shay S, Stallings K (1993) Institute for nursing excellence: a retention model. *J Cont Educ Nurs* **24**(2): 66–8

Shulman LS (1986) Those who understand: knowledge growth in teaching. *Educ Res* **15**: 4–14

Sockett HJ (1987) Has Shulman got the strategy right? *Harvard Educ Rev* **57**: 208–19

Titchen A, McIntyre D (1993) A Phenomenological Approach to Qualitative Data Analysis in Nursing Research. In: *Changing Nursing Practice through Action Research*. Report no 6, National Institute for Nursing Centre for Practice. Development and Research, Oxford

Wells HG (1987) The Country of the Blind. In: *The Complete Short Stories of H G Wells*. A & C Black (Publishers) Ltd, London

Chapter 3

The influence of autonomy and authority on nursing expertise

This chapter looks at a number of factors that are central to the development of nursing expertise. As nurses strive for excellence they need to be aware of the complex nature of expertise development. It does not develop in a vacuum and issues to do with autonomy and authority, advocacy, assertiveness and empowerment all need to be considered.

Critical incidents drawn from a study of expert nursing are used here to illustrate how these issues influenced the practice of nurses (Conway, 1995) (see Chapter 2). Many of the incidents demonstrate that expert nurses have extended and advanced their practice into areas which were previously the doctors' province.

Nursing autonomy

Autonomy means 'self-government, independence' (Oxford Paperback Dictionary). As nurses move from the role of doctors' handmaidens to independent, self-directed practitioners questions arise as to when it is legitimate for them to make autonomous decisions and when it is not.

Many nurses are extending their practice and integrating medical tasks within a nursing framework. Some are acting as autonomous practitioners on occasions. While autonomy may be but a step on the road to professionalisation, it is not to say that this journey is without problems. In particular, while experienced nurses may have the knowledge to reach decisions about patient care, they often lack the authority to follow these through in an autonomous manner.

Authority

Lack of authority

The following examples explore some of the tensions and conflicts that occur when nurses do not have the necessary authority to alter a patient care situation. An expert nurse from a coronary care unit with many years of experience described a scenario which illustrates some of the difficulties she encountered in relation to lack of authority.

'A 58-year-old ... male was admitted with an acute inferior myocardial infarction ...I noted that the patient's cardiac monitor was displaying a broad QRS complex with two P waves for every QRS and a constant P-R interval. I made the diagnosis of Type II AV block, nothing extraordinary about this. I summoned medical help. The doctor suggested that the abnormal rhythm should be observed further, with no immediate intervention.

I protested, ...that in my opinion, this was a very dangerous rhythm and could result in the demise of my patient within minutes. My rationale for intervention was that without a prophylactic pacemaker, the patient was at risk of sudden cardiac arrest. The doctor insisted that in his professional judgement, there was only a case to proceed in the event of the patient arresting. ...The doctor walked away, so I now prepared myself for the inevitable ...Behold 45 minutes later the patient developed cardiac standstill and now the pacemaker was being inserted into the heart's cavity while the resuscitation procedure was being performed. This makes the insertion of the pacemaker both difficult and hazardous. The patient did survive — but it was a catastrophic episode which should not have happened and needn't have happened if I had been listened to.'

The nurse's sense of frustration is evident in this scenario. While she had the knowledge and experience to diagnose that a potentially life-threatening situation was imminent, she was unable at the time to do anything about it. Although the nurse wanted to act as an advocate for her patient, the barriers posed by the hierarchical doctor-nurse relationship prevented this.

If nurses are to develop autonomous roles they need to feel supported by management. Unfortunately such support appears to be the exception rather than the rule. An expert Intensive Care Unit (ITU) nurse describes an incident where her authority was challenged not by doctors but by nursing management.

'We were very busy ...on ITU [with] lots of critically ill patients ...one of the patients coned ...and was going down to theatre for organ harvesting and there is a lot of organising in that. My manager thought that once the patient was brain dead, then they would not require much care and the nurse could be cancelled for the following shift. I was told to cancel a bank nurse that we had booked for the late shift and I refused to do so ...When the manager came down and saw the bank nurse, I was pulled up again for it, but I felt I justified my position. I felt that as the clinical expert I was there to tell the manager the

needs of my patients, which would reflect on the number
of staff at the time. ...It seemed as if all the manager could
see was this patient who was not moving, going on a bed
to theatre for his life to be ended and she did not seem
prepared to see beyond that. There is an awful lot of care
needed for the relatives. Had I not had the bank nurse I
feel I would have taken the incident further, but as it
happened the incident fizzled out.'

This was a very moving scenario. The expert nurse was
attempting to deal with the imminent death of her patient, a
young man, younger than herself. She used all her skill and
knowledge to enable the relatives of this young man to come
to terms with his death and with donating their son's organs.
Into this sensitive and most demanding situation intruded
the manager. The callousness of the manager's position as
perceived by the expert nurse — 'It seemed as if all the
manager could see was this patient who was not moving,
going on bed to theatre, for his life to be ended and she did
not seem prepared to see beyond that' — is almost beyond
belief. This incident raises issues to do with assertiveness,
advocacy, resources, indeed common humanity. Lack of
resources has often been quoted by nurses as the reason why
holistic care is not given, but in this example the reality in
terms of life and death is readily apparent. Issues of
conflicting values and lack of support by management are
apparent here. What is also readily evident is that the
manager and the expert nurse had very different criteria
when it came to providing care. In discussion the expert
nurse felt that:

'As nurses go higher up in management, they tell you that
their concern is the budget.'

Ambiguity of authority

Some expert nurses demonstrated knowledge through their actions which was not formally acknowledged either by medical staff or by the organisation that employed them. An expert nurse from an accident and emergency (A & E) department illustrates a case in point in the following example:

> 'Last night I took it on myself because of the nature of the circumstances that were prevailing (the A & E was very busy) to get these patients in, [and] seen in X-ray as opposed to being brought in and waiting for a medical officer, who was definitely tied up somewhere else, genuinely tied up ...What the medical officer wants is the patient and an X-ray if necessary, so that they can assess the two at the same time. So my aim was to see the patient and send them off to X-ray which I did but I have to tell you that by rights ...I am not allowed to do that.'

This expert nurse identified that he was not normally allowed to order X-rays but he felt that this 'ruling' could be broken when the department was busy and that this was acceptable to both medical and radiography staff. This situation therefore begs the question, if the expert nurse in situations of emergency can order X-rays, why can he not order X-rays at other times? Although this limited type of authority was allowed by medical staff when the department was busy, the expert identified that on other occasions he was overruled, as is apparent in this example:

> 'A female patient 82-years-old, attended the burns clinic for redressing to both lower limbs following a radiator burn. The area of full thickness in my opinion required admission, antibiotics and a total review of treatment prior to skin grafting. Following numerous discussions with the medical officer in charge my suggestions were refused. Antibiotics were commenced and the patient was

discharged back to the nursing home. The patient
developed septicaemia and died within ten days of her
discharge from clinic.'

This tragic example clearly illustrates that if it comes to a
confrontation, both the nurse and the doctor know that the
doctor's decision will hold. Although doctors and nurses are
presented as partners in the care team, the relationship is
perceived by many expert nurses as an uneven one in terms
of authority. Even though this expert nurse had many years
of experience caring for patients in A & E, the doctor chose
to ignore this nurse's requests for admission and the patient
was discharged. Possibly the patient's prognosis might still
have been as grave had she been admitted, but incidents such
as this, where expert nursing opinion is ignored without
explanation or because 'doctor knows best', serve only to
undermine the knowledge such experts have developed from
years in the practice setting.

In Conway's study, expert nurses demonstrated
considerable knowledge in their practice but this was not
always formally acknowledged. Also, although nurses were
making autonomous decisions, these were not always
recognised. Indeed, there was considerable ambiguity in
terms of authority in the way that expert nurses were treated
by doctors. While on occasions expert nurses were listened to
with respect, at other times they were ignored and overruled.
A nurse might find that one doctor would listen to her and
be guided by her while another might completely ignore her
opinion in relation to medical care. One expert nurse felt
that:

'knowing what the patient needs and then not being able
to get that provided, I think that is the most frustrating
thing that I have ever found.'

When visiting an expert nurse in theatre, this ambiguity of
authority was observed. A patient was sent down to theatre

from a coronary care unit where he had been admitted the previous day. The elderly gentleman had a suspected gastro-intestinal bleed and was there for an emergency laparotomy. The expert nurse rapidly assessed the patient's condition and took the necessary action, while simultaneously giving the patient continuous reassurance and liaising with other staff en route to the theatre. Like a director of an orchestra, the nurse issued instructions to the assembled operating team. As swiftly as the patient was transferred to the table she was instructing a nurse to change the patient's catheter bag for a urimeter. Almost simultaneously she was assisting the anaesthetist to put an arterial line into the patient's arm and at the same time kept up a reassuring dialogue with the patient.

Two student nurses looking on were now encouraged by her to be 'part of the situation'. Previously, they had looked rather lost and uneasy. As the patient was being intubated several doctors entered the theatre to observe the proceedings. The expert nurse continued to point out to the student nurses important nursing points for them to be aware of. The anaesthetist requested bloods to be sent urgently for investigation and directed his request to the expert nurse. Once again this was used as a teaching point by the expert, who took one of the students with her and showed how the blood was transferred into vacuum containers and how to complete the forms.

It was interesting to note at this juncture that this very experienced, competent expert nurse had then quickly to obtain authorisation from one of the observing doctors on the form requesting the haematological examinations. This seemed most peculiar as it was very apparent that this expert nurse had been directly involved in all aspects of this patient's care and emergency treatment, which several doctors were observing and presumably learning from. However it was accepted by all concerned that this nurse should maintain a dual role whereby on the one hand she was accepted as being capable enough to help deal with the emergency yet at the same time, she was not deemed capable of authorising the blood requests. This seemed totally incongruous and inappropriate.

Earning authority

Some scenarios demonstrate that although expert nurses may not have formal authority, they do command respect because of their knowledge and experience. An expert nurse on a coronary unit described a situation where a doctor had a problem with a pacing wire and the expert nurse diagnosed that he had inserted the pacing wire with a guard on into the cavity of the heart. The guard should have been removed before insertion.

'...I said to him that there was ... a very strong suggestion that he had left the guard over the tip of the pacing wire. "Rubbish" he said. I said to him, "Let us analyse very quickly what we have here. First of all you have been two hours in the heart, you have made no contact with the heart, the pace is still going at a rate of 30."Secondly, I told him I had checked out the pacemaker. There is a way we can test this and it is perfect...I said "What concerns me is that it is a metal guard that you have got in the heart." "How the hell could I get a stainless steel metal guard through the anti-cubital fossa and round into the inferior vena cava?" He said... "how could I go through the tricuspid valve?" I again said to him this could be done very easily, in fact more easily than without the guard on because (a) it would be heavy (b) it is stiffer. At this his whole attitude changed from being very defensive initially to becoming very humble. He said "What shall I do" and I suggested that he inform his consultant but he was adamant that would not do this... I said that I would be with him throughout the procedure. I said to him that he must not alarm the patient because the patient was conscious while all this was going on. I pointed out to him that as the heart was only beating at 30 bpm he might get away with it. What we had to do was withdraw the catheter while it was in diastole, so I kept saying diastole pull, diastole pull. As he pulled it round into the arm I compressed further down the vein so that if the guard detached at this stage it would not recirculate...Afterwards, he was as nice as could be...'

This scenario, like many of the others, raises for consideration issues such as knowledge authority and legal and ethical concerns. The expert nurse, through her knowledge and experience, was able to confront the doctor and to challenge him to listen to her diagnosis. Although initially the doctor was inclined to ignore her, she nonetheless through her demeanour and obvious knowledge base was able to convince him that she should be listened to. She clearly demonstrated knowledge of anatomy and physiology, and of how to read an image of the inside of the heart on an image intensifier. Her diagnostic ability was instrumental in influencing the doctor into taking alternative actions. When the doctor realised the seriousness of the situation then, and only then, was he prepared to listen to the expert nurse. Almost implicit in the action is the nurse acting as a partner with the doctor and of the doctor being in some sense saved by the nurse, as if the nurse was acting as an advocate for the doctor. What is not addressed in this scenario is the nature of the relationship between the nurse and the patient, and issues to do with patient information.

An expert nurse from an anaesthetic recovery area provides another clear example of the need to earn authority.

'All of the patients that we go and see who are having post-op analgesia, we go and see them on the ward and assess them and talk over [our findings] with the anaesthetist. Now he may think that the patient is suitable for patient-controlled analgesia. When I have gone along and found that some of these patients seem unsuitable, I would discuss with him the reasons why I think they are unsuitable. Usually he will say "Trust you to pick that up, and yes, I agree with you".

We had one lady ...she was a very highly strung lady who told the anaesthetist that she was quite happy to have patient-controlled analgesia but when I asked her if she understood how to use it, it was quite clear that she did not understand how to use it and she could not cope with it. We did try her with it back on the ward and she had the ward in uproar screaming! Oh, she was dreadful ...so now he does listen to me and if I say I don't think this patient is suitable, he will say "Yes you are right". Sometimes you have to prove yourself before they will listen to you.'

This expert nurse makes an excellent point that 'sometimes you have to prove yourself before they will listen to you', but this seems a ludicrous position if expert nurses have to keep doing this with each new doctor to their area.

Informal authority

In many areas the role of the expert nurse vis-à-vis the doctor is not clear cut and nurses extend their practice in an informal manner. Many specialist expert nurses have advanced their knowledge to the extent that they give advice and guidance to medical staff. Expert nurses frequently bridge the gap between consultants and junior medical staff. An expert oncology nurse described her role in recommending medication for patients undergoing chemotherapy:

'Other than signing the prescription I recommend the drug to the houseman because I have got more knowledge generally than the houseman. I have more knowledge on the chemotherapy drugs themselves, on the administration of chemotherapy and on drugs associated with chemotherapy like the anti-emetic drugs ...I expect a houseman to listen to me because I do have more knowledge than he has ...generally they are very good. The house officers are only looking after them [patients] for three months at a time so I know the patients when they don't and I know the drug regimes whereas generally they don't because, unfortunately, we don't have a registrar for Haematology so there is nobody between the senior house-officer and the consultant so generally I fill that gap.'

Expert nurses who work in specialist areas become familiar with the usual regimes and treatments carried out. Also, in areas such as oncology, where patients can be receiving treatment for many years, nurses get to know patients and their responses in a way that is not possible for medical staff who only stay a few months (Porter, 1991 citing Hughes, 1988).

Informal authority and responsibility

The study showed that expert nurses who had informal authority were mindful of their responsibilities and valued the freedom they were given by medical staff.

'A lot of it boils down to the authority they [the doctors] have given us practising that way. Obviously, if we didn't work in a unit where we have the co-operation of the medical staff to allow us to practise like that then we couldn't but they have given us the freedom to develop those skills.'

During a visit to a post-cardiac surgery unit an expert nurse discussed her views on extending the nursing role in her area and the issues that arise from this:

'I know that we are very privileged, there are very few places like our area and we do recognise that. Junior staff can be a problem ...we have to teach them that this is not normal and what they see me doing is not something they will be aspiring to do in six months or next year but in five, six, seven [or] eight years. You have to actually work very very hard to help very junior staff realise the scope of practice that we undertake and [to] have the insight into their own limitations...

We don't have junior anaesthetic cover in the unit so if we do have patients ventilated it is up to the senior nursing staff to make any adjustments that are needed to the ventilators. Now, that is very unusual. They don't do that in the general intensive care unit here and there are very, very few places I am sure that allow nurses that freedom. So if you get a junior D grade and they see us doing it... and they look and they think "I know what to do, I'll do the ventilator"and they don't realise that it is an exceptional thing we are allowed to do, not normal, you have to say to them you may well be right ...[but] you are still not going to do it, I will do it .. you don't have the freedom to go and adjust the ventilator as you think fit or turn the ionotropes up if the blood pressure falls or anything really like that.'

In this nurse's unit authority for activities such as setting ventilators has passed from the medical staff to senior nursing staff. In turn, these expert nurses ensure that other nurses have sufficient knowledge and experience before they too are allowed to extend their roles in this way.

Formal extension of nursing practice and authority

In some areas, nurses have been given formal authority to carry out certain tasks previously the province of doctors through the use of protocols and by having specific activities written into their contracts. An expert diabetic specialist describes how this works in her situation.

'We do change dosage of both oral agents and insulin and it is written into our contract. We recommend to GPs ..I have just done it this morning. A patient who was seen two months ago as a newly diagnosed diabetic ...is not responding to diet-only and he needs some help. So I phoned the GP's surgery this morning and spoke with them ...and I have suggested that perhaps we ought to start some Metformin... sometimes we will ring GPs and say that perhaps they might be better not on the one oral agent but that they might have a better response to another or it might be that they are already on an oral agent and that we could add Metformin or we do very often ring and say "look your patient just isn't helping on the oral agent. I think we are at the stage to consider insulin".'

In other areas specialist nurses are also advancing their practice into territory previously the province of medical staff. An expert total parenteral nutrition (TPN) nurse explained that the experience she had gained when working in ITU had enabled her to be innovative in relation to her present post in caring for patients who undergo total parenteral nutrition. She believed that she could improve the service she provided by taking on the responsibility for inserting TPN lines herself. This is a procedure normally carried out in theatre where a doctor inserts a tube (called a line) into a vein and guides the line around into the patient's heart. The patient is fed with liquid food through this line. This expert decided to approach the senior surgeon with a view to receiving training to insert lines for TPN feeding.

'I was quite expecting the director of surgery to fall over backwards when I suggested it.'

Nursing management were extremely supportive and she commented that without this support such an innovation would not have been possible. In terms of success

'...the way we are doing it, we are keeping patients out of theatre; we are reducing their anaesthetic risk because there is none and they are able to have the lines put in on the ward that they are familiar with, with nurses around them that they know and they just feel very much more confident about the whole thing, which has to be good for them.'

This expert reported that the infection rate had been dramatically reduced. Several important issues underlie this nurse's extension of her role. She has demonstrated that she is capable of acting in an autonomous manner when given the authority to do so. Instead of acting as an assistant to a doctor while he makes the incision and threads the TPN line into the *vena cava* (a vein entering the heart), she carried out from beginning to end this invasive procedure. The author observed her inserting a TPN line, while she showed two doctors how to do it. Her quiet confidence and composure was impressive, and there was no doubting that she was viewed with respect.

Conclusion

If nurses with knowledge and experience are to fully utilise their abilities and act in an autonomous manner for the good of patients, then it is desirable that this is formally acknowledged by all concerned. Protocols provide opportunities for nurses to extend their practice in this manner. Protocols may also resolve the ambiguity of authority that many experts are exposed to. How can any nurse develop confidence in his/her practice if on one occasion they are allowed to carry out a certain activity but on another they are censured for doing the same thing? Nurses who demonstrate extensive knowledge bases in relation to patient care do not need their confidence undermining by expecting them to pay lip service to outdated hierarchies and needless bureaucracy.

References

Conway JE (1995) *Expert Nursing Knowledge as an Evolutionary Process*. Unpublished PhD thesis, University of Warwick, Coventry

Porter S (1991) A participant observation study of power relations between nurses and doctors in a general hospital. *J Adv Nurs* **16**: 728–35

.

Chapter 4

Doctor-nurse relationships

This chapter examines the doctor-nurse relationship in terms of its influence on knowledge use and development in the practice setting. Some effects of this relationship have been described elsewhere (Stein, 1967; Lubin and Gething, 1983; Murray, 1986; Stein *et al*, 1990; Sweet and Norman, 1995). However, its impact on the development of expert knowledge has not previously been identified. Historically while nurses post-Nightingale were not quite seen as slaves, they were nonetheless seen as little more than servants by medical staff. Within such relationships a type of benign paternalism operated. Gender differences with doctors (mainly male) and nurses (female) further reinforced power differences between the two:

> *'The relationship between the doctor and the nurse is a special one, based on mutual respect and interdependence, steeped in history and stereotyped in popular culture'* (Stein *et al*, 1990).

This relationship was described as long ago as the 1960s by Stein (1967). He presented the interactions that resulted from this relationship as a form of game playing:

'Nurses were to be bold, have initiative and be responsible for making important recommendations, while at the same time they had to seem passive... Thus, nurses needed to communicate their recommendations [to doctors] without appearing to make them' (Stein *et al, 1990*).

This is seen as a reflection of the relationship of men and women in society:

'Patriarchy can be seen in the doctor-nurse relationship by drawing parallels between the husband and wife in the family, with the nurse looking after the physical and emotional environment, whilst the doctor decided what the really important work was, and how it was to be done' (Oakley, 1984; Abbott and Wallace, 1990 cited by Sweet and Norman, 1995).

The relationship has also been examined in terms of social roles and power relationships (Sweet and Norman, 1995).

At long last changes are occurring in this relationship. In the last five to ten years, as nursing has moved into higher education, considerable realignment of boundaries has started to take place. As nurses become better educated they become more able to challenge their medical colleagues should the need arise.

The doctor-nurse relationship has a direct influence on the way nurses develop and use knowledge in the clinical setting (Conway, 1995). In addition, this relationship has strong links with the type of care given to patients. Some relationships are very positive and nurses feel valued and supported. Others are far less satisfactory and show a form of oppression by medical staff in relation to nurses. The consequences of such relationships have to be thought through. As the boundaries between nursing and medicine become more and more blurred we must ensure that suitable relationships are in place to support advances into what was previously medical territory.

Devising strategies to ensure positive relationships

In terms of doctor-nurse relationships many nurses see themselves as being the flexible ones. They also see themselves as being the ones who strive for positive relationships with their medical colleagues. An experienced nurse from a gastro-enterology unit identified that:

'The trouble is here and certainly in theatre you seem to work with a lot of little egos that all have to be pampered to. They are not easy. I think sometimes it is a bit like watching a creche... Probably working in a creche would be a lot easier. I bear in mind how certain people like things; one will like this on such a day, one will like something else on another day. I go along with it up to a point, up to a point...'

In terms of the doctor-nurse relationship expert nurses perceive themselves as being pro-active and negotiating in a diplomatic manner. This can be seen in the next example where an expert nurse from a surgical area described the time and effort that she put into attempting to establish positive doctor-nurse relationships in her area:

'While initially I think consultants are extremely or can be extremely threatening, particularly to more junior staff nurses and anybody else, I have worked very, very hard to get over that. I haven't managed it completely, I don't think I will ever manage it completely, but I have been influential in improving things a lot... The way I did it was to stick my neck out to some extent with the consultants to say this is me, this is what I believe in, here I am. As expected, like dogs to a bone, they worry it and give it a hard time until it does not get worried any more. They gave me a hard time to begin with. I was expecting them to and I stood my ground and I just said fine, yes... I conceded on a lot of things... but I never conceded the whole way. I did all the consultant ward rounds but I always insisted that the nurses looking after the patients were included as well and then, gradually, as the consultants have got used to it, I have taken a step backwards... its not [now] such an issue that I have to be there.'

While this relationship may not have been ideal to start with, this nurse used strategies to ensure that, gradually, change was able to take place. She also identified that her concern for positive relationships with medical staff was perhaps influential in determining her own research interests and studies. I asked her if she had deliberately chosen a human biology degree, specialising in the same area as the speciality she worked in because it would improve her credibility with the surgeons with whom she worked.

'Possibly, ...I suppose having a human biology degree, particularly if you tell them you are doing a dissertation on [a specific] cancer and they are ...surgeons [in that speciality] and you go and interview them, and show that you know what you are talking about has to lend you some credibility and kudos and I suppose if I was ...being completely honest, I could even say that might have had some influence on why I chose to do it. I don't wish to become a doctor, I wish to bridge the gap between the two professions and work for us working together for the patients.'

Clearly, this nurse put considerable energy and commitment into developing positive relationships with the medical staff. She devised unique strategies to ensure that nursing was respected by the medical consultants in her area and that nursing initiatives were accepted by them.

Monitoring and correcting junior doctors

Experienced nurses often spent considerable time correcting and monitoring junior doctors in their areas. This function was not 'officially recognised'. Medical consultants might, on an informal basis, tell junior doctors to make sister or charge nurse their best friend while the juniors were working in the unit. But on a more formal recognitional level, it was evident that the monitoring and diagnostic element of the nurse's role vis-à-vis junior doctors was not acknowledged. An expert nurse from an ITU describes her role with regard to such monitoring:

'I think correcting doctors happens all the time. The number of times in ITU that we have saved patients' lives through stopping doctors from doing something, or from telling them to do something, is too numerous to count. I think because we are a specialised unit, the doctors tend to have a lot of respect for the nursing staff. Sometimes I can't believe the number of patients that would have come to harm if we had not intervened and I wonder how many things have happened in the past that we do not know about? They often forget to write the right dose of Ranitidine or they have forgotten to write it altogether, or they change a vent [ventilator] setting. It takes you years to get to know certain ventilators, all the little things about them, and they will still come along and change a setting and walk away and they have done the wrong thing, or they haven't entered it properly. There is always something not right and you pick it up as the nurse caring for that patient. I will approach the doctor and ask them if they understand the ventilator and they tend to say that it is not very complicated, when it is and they think they understand them, when they really do not... A lot of the nurses' policies are directed at checking that the doctors have done things at the correct time, and correctly.'

Such monitoring forms part of the hidden world of nursing. It is initiated as a safeguard for patients, yet recognised by few outside of the care setting (Lubin and Gething, 1983). From a deep sense of responsibility to the patient, nurses perceive the need for such monitoring yet this is not acknowledged formally by medical staff or management. This nurse also discussed the difficulties she had encountered when her knowledge of how to deal with a cardiac arrest was greater than that of the junior doctor dealing with the arrest situation:

'Each arrest is different and it is very difficult when you are at an arrest and you see junior doctors trying to cope and you know what drugs the patient needs or you know what should be done and you have to bite your tongue and you think to yourself, "I might make a fool of myself if I am wrong", but if the patient's life is at stake I speak up. What I tend to do is draw up the injections and I say "I have got the adrenaline here" you know, do it tactfully. Or I would say "I have got the calcium ready for when you want it" and they would go "Oh yes, I'll give some calcium". Some of them will say to get some soda bicarb, but that is out now, ...so I say "haven't you read the research," or "haven't you been to the cardio pulmonary resuscitation lecture?" because every junior doctor should go but they don't go.'

This is a good example of how complex knowledge usage by expert nurses is. The expert starts by identifying that each arrest is different, therefore it is not sufficient to have a list of instructions to follow. Rather, knowledge of principles has to be applied to differing situations. It is also likely that such scenarios, because of their uniqueness, will require the expert nurse to be able to reflect-in-action (Schon, 1987) so that each unique case can be responded to in an appropriate manner. There is also evidence in the scenario that the expert nurse felt that she had to play the doctor-nurses game (Stein *et al*, 1990) where she pretends for the doctor's benefit that he has thought of something that was really her suggestion. This area of inequality of relationships between doctors and nurses caused considerable difficulties on occasions:

> 'A lot of the doctors do not do the correct compressions and constantly... massage far too quick so they are pushing on an empty heart. I tell them sometimes... It is different if it is a nurse, I do not hesitate then. If it is a doctor that I know, I would tell him if he was doing compressions wrong but if it is a doctor I do not know and I'm not sure what rank he is, I'm a bit dubious.'

While the expert nurse in this scenario had the knowledge to know how CPR resuscitation should be carried out, because of the hierarchical relationship between doctors and nurses, she was reluctant to challenge doctors she did not know. She felt that she needed to handle the relationship between herself and the doctors carefully. She was prepared to tell doctors when they were not carrying out cardiac compressions correctly but she presented this as conditional: she did this if it was a doctor that she knew. It is a cause for disquiet that this very experienced and expert ITU nurse felt that if the doctor was unknown to her or if she was unsure of his rank, then she was dubious about telling him when he was doing cardiac compressions incorrectly. In such a situation, it is possible that this hierarchical, unequal relationship could lead to an unsuccessful resuscitation effort and thus the death of the patient. This is not intended as criticism of this expert, rather as a testimonial to the strength of the inhibiting factors that the expert nurse felt were on her when it came to working with doctors.

Medical support for development of the nursing role

In some specialist areas nurses have been encouraged by doctors to develop the nurse's role and integrate medical tasks and responsibilities into it. An expert nurse from a post-cardiac unit identified that making decisions previously made by doctors was not always easy and that many factors had to be considered. Nurses in the area in which she worked had been able to extend their practice not only because they had extended their knowledge bases but also because the doctors were prepared to give these nurses the authority to do so. In the following example, she highlights some of the factors involved in making decisions about extubating patients post-cardiac surgery:

> '...99% of the time [patients are] intubated and ventilated when they come back to the unit so if a patient wakes up you then have to go through a process of making the decision of whether to sedate the patient and keep them ventilated or ...take them off the ventilator and that is entirely a nursing decision as to whether you take them off the ventilator, allow them to breathe and then make the decision to extubate them and that has no longer got anything to do with our medical staff; that is purely a nursing decision.'

In this particular unit experienced nurses had considerably extended their roles into what had been traditionally medical areas. The knowledge base of this expert had been developed over the years through both theory and practice, thus facilitating this process.

Taking risks

Decision-making involves a degree of risk taking. Nurses have to be able to weigh up situations and then take a calculated decision as to the specific action which should be taken. This often involves an element of risk taking. The expert described some of the factors that she considered during such situations:

> 'Sometimes it is very easy; it is very clear what you are going to do but then you get the patient that it is not so clear and not so easy and I think then again you are drawing on your knowledge, your past experience and the likely effect of your action or inaction on that patient... Quite often you have to take a risk and you have to weigh up if that is a risk worth taking as to whether or not you would extubate someone and sort of go with it... Sometimes it can be quite difficult to decide whether to extubate or resedate someone and I think again it is quite an easy way of showing people who have got the ability to actually work through all the different indicators and make the decisions of what is most appropriate. We either go for a rapid extubation or a weaning, we adjust all our ventilator fittings ourselves so... we would not even tell the doctors. We don't, we don't even tell them, or if we needed to sedate we would choose which sedation to use and we would start that ourselves...'

The nurses in this area had successfully extended their nursing role. They had been able to do this because they had been given the authority to do so. They were sufficiently assertive to be able to take calculated risks when the occasion demanded.

A great deal of knowledge underpins this type of action. In order to prescribe medication, the nurses have to have an understanding of pharmacology and the ways drugs are metabolised in the body both in a normal person and in a person who has undergone cardiac surgery. Side-effects and contra-indications also need to be known so that the nurse is making judgements based on a sound knowledge base. In terms of setting a ventilator a number of knowledge bases would be required. The nurse needs a knowledge of the parameters of normality. In terms of the patient's condition both physical and psychological factors have to be considered post-operatively. Knowledge is required of normal and abnormal respiration and of the cardiovascular system. Managing ventilators correctly is about much more than developing a skill; it is about developing extensive knowledge bases on which the skill is built.

In other areas the readjustment of boundaries between medicine and nursing is taking place much more gradually and in an informal manner. This type of transition seems to have more to do with nurses taking authority rather than doctors delegating it.

Informal adjustment of the boundaries of practice

A nurse from a medical unit explained that in his area the boundaries between medicine and nursing were not always clear cut. This example illustrates the informal authority that nurses take on occasions and that this is accepted by medical staff:

'I occasionally do make decisions previous, you know make decisions and tell the doctor [later that] I have done it and more often than not they are happy with that decision... We haven't properly explored, say, things like nurse prescribing but in effect there are members of the staff and I am certainly one of them, who would occasionally give a fairly limited number of drugs without asking the doctor first; that is less of a formal agreement and more of an understood agreement. But I suppose that comes more into the realm of game playing at the moment, but I think that will be more formalised... We are developing but maybe the formal barriers are not readjusting.'

This example illustrates that on occasions nurses are prepared to take decisions that they do not always have the authority to make. This highlights the need for protocols and procedures for such decisions. As boundaries alter and readjust, it is essential that supporting protocols are developed so that such nurses are not out on a limb and possibly subject to disciplinary action.

Experience and authority

Nurses occasionally direct doctors' actions. The next example illustrates this points clearly:

'We had a patient who had been out of theatre for about an hour after cardiac surgery. We were just about to extubate him, the nurse looking after him had sat him up and his gases were good and we were literally ...about to cut the ET tube tapes and take the tubes out when his chest drains just filled with blood and it just poured down the drains and his blood pressure went from 140 to 60.

I just remembered this is something that I have seen before and what had happened was that one of his grafts had actually come off and the only way to do anything about it is to re-open that patient there and then. I just dived outside the door and there was a poor registrar who had just been on the unit five days and I just said you just have to open that patient's chest, and he had never actually done it himself, and I said you just have to cut the stitches and take the wires out while we got the surgeon back...

I just remember having to tell this registrar over and over again "just cut the stitches and take the wires out".. His next question was "but he is not anaesthetised." I said "it does not matter, he is going to be unconscious in a minute," by which time he was unconscious because his pressure was so low and... eventually we had three different lines going into this gentleman to replace his circulating volume and by the time we opened his chest his drain bottles were full, three litres in the bottle, the rest of his circulating volume was in his pericardium really. We got the end of the graft sewn back on and we left him that night ventilated and we really did not think he would do very well. I was most surprised.. to see him next morning sitting up eating his cornflakes!' (Expert nurse, post-cardiac ITU).

The nurse in this scenario demonstrates how through experience she was able to diagnose the patient's condition and the absolute necessity for immediate action. Her insistence on prompt action resulted in a positive patient outcome. A synthesis of experiential knowledge and assertive ability ensured that the patient received the necessary treatment on this occasion.

Nursing knowledge and junior doctors

Discussions with many of the experts studied revealed that they felt in specific areas nurses were more knowledgeable than junior doctors (Lubin and Gething, 1983). In the following example, an expert nurse from a surgical area described her feelings about the knowledge nurses had in her field:

'...I have got staff nurses who have been here for two, three or four years.. [They] are more knowledgeable about pre- and post-operative care than junior doctors. They are not as knowledgeable as consultants are... but in terms of managing the majority of patients through our ward the senior experienced nurses are teaching young doctors how to do it.'

When asked to specify what particular types of knowledge this expert nurse was referring to, she replied:

'Everything; assessing, nutritional support, psychological information... not breaking bad news but giving patients information about their diagnosis. I remember I interviewed a consultant in my study and I said "What do you feel about information giving, do you get a sense [that] there are certain things that certain disciplines should talk about and those are boundaries that should be maintained?"... We had quite a long talk about nurses giving patients information about their diagnosis [and] prognosis. He said "to be honest... I have no problem with your senior nurses doing that, you know more, [or] as much as I do about it". But I have a problem if I go to another ward or department. So you have to take it on an individual basis, but in essence there is the recognition that some nurses do have that knowledge base and experience that is being used in managing patients' whole care, probably more effectively and satisfactorily from the patient's point of view, not necessarily from the doctor's. They don't always like it when you steal their thunder — well some do, because they are not very good at telling patients bad news and they are quite relieved that nurses have done it and have probably done it quite well and sensitively.'

The consultant was prepared to acknowledge that in some areas the expert nurse knows as much as, if not more than, he does. Such a view is still uncommon. The consultant was also prepared to acknowledge that nurses in this area were likely to have the knowledge to cope with diagnosis and prognostic information-giving, but he also emphasised that this did not apply to all areas. The expert nurse explained:

> 'It is new territory, exploring diagnosis... but so often the questions that are asked are within nursing's domain to answer and they are not within the surgeon's or physician's necessarily and they [surgeons] are not interested in some of those questions like "How regular will my bowels be? What kind of diet should I take?" They are not really interested.
>
> The [surgeons] are interested if the cancer is there and what kind of operative technique they might use, so it does complement very well working together... quite often, certainly in the early days, I would have junior staff nurses alongside me for these conversations. They would come and observe some of my interactions with clients and we talked about it afterwards. I know when I [can] take an observer into a situation and when I can't. There are some conversations where I am so strung up I can't. It is bad enough being in the conversation, never mind having someone watch you with your umms and ahhs, struggling with it.'

Clearly the expert nurse felt confident to push forward the boundaries of her practice into the realms of diagnosis exploration. She was mindful of the medical role in this process, but appreciated that, in reality, many of the worries and problems that patients asked about were within nursing's domain. She also clearly demonstrated a reflective approach to her practice in deciding when it was appropriate for learners to be observing and when it was not. Her open admission that sometimes she felt she would not cope with an observer also reflected personal insight and awareness of her own strengths and weakness in a non-judgmental but assertive manner.

Developing assertiveness

The transition from being a doctor's assistant to becoming an independent practitioner requires a readjustment in decision-making ability. An expert TPN nurse explained that having confidence in her own ability rather than being directed by a doctor was something that developed over time. In terms of expertise, as well as the importance of a supportive culture, she felt that it was important not to be too self-critical and suggested that nurses should:

> 'Treat each patient as an individual and when something goes wrong to use that as a learning exercise, not to be too self-critical.'

While this sentiment makes sense, for many this would be almost impossible. As long as nurses work in environments where to get something wrong is unacceptable, then practice will remain defensive. These nurses will struggle to 'cover their backs' and ensure that they cannot be criticised for anything. If nurses are to continue to develop their practice and to extend into the realms of medical tasks, then they need to know that they are supported. Also, nurses need to be encouraged to learn from negative experiences as well as positive ones.

Conclusion

The yoke of history is not always easily thrown off. The effects of socialising nurses into believing that they were subordinate to doctors cannot be altered over night. Higher education may go some way to bringing about change but outdated practices at the bedside also need to change.If nurses are monitoring junior doctors' actions then this needs to be explicitly recognised by medical staff (Lubin and Gething, 1983). Environments need to be created at ward level where nurses feel safe to develop their practice. They need to feel secure enough to use their own judgements and make informed choices even if this means on occasions taking informed risks. If nurses feel oppressed by medical staff, they will not be able to do this.

References

Conway JE (1995) *Expert Nursing Knowledge as an Evolutionary Process*. Unpublished PhD Thesis. University of Warwick, Coventry

Lubin J, Gething L (1983) RNs as teachers of junior doctors. *Aus J Adv Nurs* **10**(2): 3–9

Murray FJ (1986) The manoeuvring continues in the doctor-nurse game. *Med World News* **March 10**: 81–97

Schon DA (1987) *Educating the Reflective Practitioner*. Jossey-Bass, London

Stein LI (1967) The doctor nurse game. *Arch Gen Psychiatry* **16**(6): 699–703

Stein LI, Watts DT, Howell T (1990) Sounding board: the doctor nurse game revisited. *New Eng J Med* **322**(8): 546–9

Sweet SJ, Norman IJ (1995) The nurse-doctor relationship: a selective literature review. *J Adv Nurs* **22**: 165–70

Chapter 5

Practical nursing knowledge

This chapter considers the nature of practical nursing knowledge. While historically theoretical knowledge was valued in nursing, practice was seen as being based on theory derived from outside the clinical setting. Theory and practice were seen as separate entities with little relationship between the two. Consequently, a theory-practice gap developed (McCaugherty, 1992a; 1992b). It is only in the last ten to fifteen years that a re-appraisal of knowledge found in practice (Benner, 1984) and, more widely, of the concept of professional knowledge itself (Schon, 1983; 1987) has taken place.

Early descriptions of nursing knowledge are still useful and Carper's (1978) fundamental patterns of knowing provide a starting point for considerations of nursing practical knowledge.

What is practical nursing knowledge?

Table 5.1: Carper's (1978) Fundamental Patterns of Knowing in Nursing

Empirics	The Science of Nursing
Aesthetics	The Art of Nursing
Personal Knowledge	
Ethics	The Moral Component

Empirical knowledge can be seen as providing a scientific research base to nursing:

> *'There is a critical need for knowledge about the empirical world, that is systematically organised into general laws and theories for the purpose of describing, explaining and predicting phenomena of special concern to the discipline of nursing'* (Carper, 1978: 14).

Aesthetics is described as being concerned with the 'Art of Nursing'. Wiedenbach, cited by Carper (1978: 16–7), suggests that the art of nursing is:

> *'...made visible through actions taken to provide whatever the patient requires to restore or extend his ability to cope with the demands of his situation.'*

Artistry is the taken-for-granted aspect of practice and has received scant recognition, particularly in academic terms. Under the heading of aesthetics Carper (1978: 17) also identifies empathy as 'an important mode in the aesthetic pattern of knowing'.

The personal knowledge component is 'the most problematic, the most difficult to master and teach' (Carper, 1978: 18). This component represents the knowledge evident in nurse-patient relationships. It is concerned with interpersonal processes and involves interactions, relationships and transactions. The phrase 'therapeutic use of self', which has become increasingly prominent in the literature, implies that the way in which nurses view themselves and the patient/client is of primary concern in any therapeutic relationship.

The fourth and final practice of knowing concerns the ethical dimension of nursing practice:

> *'The ethical pattern of knowing in nursing requires an understanding of different philosophical positions regarding what is good, what ought to be desired, what is right, of different ethical frameworks devised for dealing with the complexities of moral judgements; and of various orientations to the notion of obligation'* (Carper, 1978:21).

Benner's (1984) seminal work provides the next milestone in terms of identifying nursing practical knowledge. Focusing on the proposition that perceptual awareness is central to good nursing judgement and that this begins with vague hunches, she contends that the knowledge embedded in clinical practice accrues over time (Benner, 1984). Her work focuses on nurses' discretionary judgement used in clinical situations. She addresses the risky, situation-specific decisions that are usually covered up, but that nurses face in their practice every day. The central premise of her work is that:

> *'...expertise develops when the clinician tests and refines propositions, hypotheses and principle-based expectations in actual practice situations'* (Benner, 1984:3).

She identifies six types of practical knowledge (1) graded qualitative distinctions (2) common meanings, (3) assumptions, expectations and sets, (4) paradigm cases and personal knowledge, (5) maxims and (6) unplanned practices. Nurses acquire knowledge as they move from novice to expert through a five stage sequence. Benner has set the scene for a new awareness and appreciation of practical nursing knowledge.

In her work which examines the practice of expert nurses (Conway, 1995 and Chapter 2 of this book), Conway found that numerous knowledge bases were used by expert nurses. These were often used simultaneously and are thus called simultaneous complex reasoning. Here an expert nurse illustrates this synthesising of several knowledge bases:

> 'We can't pretend that some of the things we do can only be done by registered nurses...I am very proud that 12 years after starting nursing, I am still giving essential nursing care and I see myself as being quite good at cleaning teeth and washing people and things like that. Of course, the actual mechanical activities of doing those things can be done by all sorts of people, can be done by unqualified people, can be done by lay people... [However,] I can do this at the same time as giving drugs, taking observations, building relationships and participating in the management of the hospital. Standing up for nursing in the inter-professional debate, planning discharges, co-operating with physiotherapists, occupational therapists ...I can do that all at the same time and that is the specialness of being a professional nurse' (Expert nurse).

Competency approaches

Because of its complexity, nursing knowledge does not lend itself to measurement by competency approaches. Indeed behaviourist models have limited value in evaluating nursing knowledge:

> *'Nursing competence involves more than knowledge and skill: also included within this domain are the*

processes of critical, creative and reflective thinking,
decision-making and problem-solving. Indeed, it may
be argued that these processes represent the main
components of nursing practice' (Fitzpatrick et al, 1992:
1214).

Simply examining the competence demonstrated by nurses
is an inadequate approach to examining nursing practical
knowledge. Values and characteristics also require attention.
It is not the task that the expert carries out that is significant,
it is the 'world view' in terms of the knowledge and attitudes
brought to the task that determines the care given. Critics of
competency approaches in higher education express concerns
that are relevant here:

'Programmes based on the functional analysis of work
roles are likely to produce teachers who are 'competent'
yet ill-equipped for further professional development,
uncritical of educational change and largely ignorant
of the wider cultural, social and political context in
which the role of teachers needs to be located. Such
teachers will be neither experts nor reflective
practitioners and will be professional in name only'
(Hyland, 1993: 130).

These insights support Conway's findings (Conway, 1995 and
Chapter 2 of this book), that expertise is about much more
than having a certain amount of subject matter knowledge.
The points Hyland (1993) makes can be applied equally well
to nursing. Indeed, expertise development is influenced by
wider social, political and cultural influences and only some
types of expertise followed a professional model.

The knowledge used by expert nurses will now be
discussed in more detail. The experts will be considered in
the categories of Technologists, Specialists, Traditionalists
and Humanistic Existentialists, as described in Chapter 2 (see
pp 15–17).

Technologists' Knowledge

Technologists demonstrated a wide variety of knowledge bases. Examples included knowledge of anatomy and physiology, pharmacology, chemotherapy, disease processes and knowledge of complications arising from conditions. Experts anticipated likely scenarios and prepared for them. They did this by considering a complex variety of 'cues' and their implications. Having decided a likely outcome, the experts then prepared for it. An expert from an ITU explained her thinking when she detected something was not quite right with a patient situation:

> 'I begin to become aware that things are not quite what they were and they could either go away or they could get worse and I just start to think, "What has he had done? What is his fluid state?" and generally do a full sweep of the patient, ...subconsciously I am thinking about his IV access, "Has he got inotropes up?" If I need to give him volume, "What lines have I got?" ...drains everything, really quickly run through all of his systems, ...just look at the monitor and work my way down quickly...'

This nurse exhibits the ability to assess a complex variety of cues. She explained:

> 'You could have a situation where you have two patients identical, who have had the same operation, who have had the same amount of fluid, the same amount of blood loss, same urine output and they have dropped their blood pressure. The one patient I might not worry about if he was very warm, very dilated, it would not worry me at all ...[however,] if the patient next door was cold, then that would worry me a lot.'

This nurse demonstrates a discriminating ability. She determines not only which factors are significant, but also when and why they are significant. She identifies the seriousness of apparently small discrepancies in a patient's condition, such as the patient being cold and she is able to detect the potential seriousness of this.

Anticipatory knowledge

In this next example, an expert anaesthetic nurse discussed the importance of anticipating events:

> 'It is anticipating all the time... you are ready before you need to be and you don't end up having to sort things out... perhaps I will just have some dopamine sitting on the side, perhaps I will have an extra syringe pump, perhaps I will have this, perhaps I will have that and then when they actually need it and they say "I will have some dopamine" it is in your syringe pump and there you are. Or if you think he might need an arterial line and you said to the anaesthetist "Will you need one" and they have said "No I don't think so"... it might be three hours before they come to theatre, ...[you] take a blood pressure and it is low and the anaesthetist will say "We will have an arterial line" but it is there, it is ready because you have anticipated you might need it.'

In this example, the expert identifies the importance of being prepared and having sufficient knowledge to be able to deal with all eventualities. Also, the importance of trusting your own judgement is apparent as opposed to merely doing what the anaesthetist specifies. The expert explained that 'You learn to take very little of what the anaesthetist says verbatim'. Her expertness is apparent in the degree of autonomy she demonstrated as opposed to preparing for situations as directed by the anaesthetist. She is much more than a pair of hands for the doctor; she is in a sense acting as another self. She also needs a knowledge of complications that may arise so that she is able to prepare for them.

Recognising early warning symptoms

In the next example, an expert from an intensive care unit
(ITU) described a situation in which she was able to pick up
early warning signals, such as the patient becoming fidgety
and restless, and was able to start considering alternative
scenarios before the student working with her was able to do
so. Not only was the expert nurse quicker at picking up 'cues'
but she was also quicker at anticipating that a chest X-ray
would be required. Information-processing was more
sophisticated, quicker and involved a decision-making
element as compared to that of the student, which involved
a slower process dependent on limited indicators and without
a decision-making or action element included:

> '...This lady... had a massive infarct (coronary thrombosis)
> ...she needed ventilating for a while and we had literally
> just extubated her the day before... she was fine sitting up
> in bed and then she started to get quite fidgety and really
> quite restless, and then her respiratory rate went up. It was
> all sorts of things like that, before you saw her saturation
> drop and by this time I was beginning to think it is
> respiratory, and I was starting to check the fluid balance,
> thinking when had the student last done a gas to check
> her oxygenation... I was beginning to think maybe she is
> going into pulmonary oedema. Her sputum was clear that
> was OK, so by this time her sats (saturations) were starting
> to drop, so I got Jacky to do a blood gas. I was already
> thinking we need an X-ray here. So by the time we got the
> doctor, I sort of decided to ring for an X-ray and they just
> said "Yes, go ahead and do it". It proved that she had got
> pulmonary oedema so we just gave her Lasix and sorted
> it out.'

Not only was the expert nurse able to differentiate between
normal and abnormal scenarios, she was also able to exclude
other possibilities. For example, she was checking the

patient's sputum to ascertain if it was blood-stained as this could indicate that a pulmonary embolism (clot in the lungs) had occurred.

Monitoring

The monitoring aspect of care provision was evident during an observation visit to an expert recovery nurse. When asked to talk through her feelings and concerns when caring for a child immediately after an operation, she presented her thoughts and actions as follows:

> 'Concerned about her airway ... looking and observing for signs of breathing ... seeing if she was breathing on her own which she was, looking at the air coming back clouding and misting up the ET tube; looking at the oxygen saturation; looking at her heart rate; if her heart rate suddenly starts to increase, wondering if she was obstructing further down the tube or whether in fact she was lightly still under the anaesthetic, which she was. Once we started to suck, she went into spasm. The anaesthetist was quite happy for me to take over and suction her and give her the oxygen. I was checking to see if she was breath holding which children sometimes do, and then measuring her respiratory rate which was 28; her saturation was low at first but the sensor was not picking it up properly and with an adjustment it shot up to 95. I was quite happy with her.'

In this example, the expert demonstrated not only complex abilities to deal with and think of many differing things at the same time, she also demonstrated specialist knowledge derived from practice about how children sometimes breath hold post-operatively. She also, in common with other expert technologists showed a healthy distrust of the sensor, when she identified that it was not recording the oxygen saturation satisfactorily, and was content to trust her own assessment of the child's condition.

Diagnosing

Technologists used a synthesis of subject matter knowledge and experience to inform their practice. They were constantly diagnosing. They did this by considering complex and varied factors often in a changing situation and then coming to a judgement. An expert coronary care unit (CCU) nurse talked through her thought processes when a patient described his symptoms to her:

> 'The way he described his symptoms is very typical, that [mention of the] internal aspect of the arm where the pain was, is highly suspect because of the nervous distribution from the heart. The cardiac plexus actually tracks down the arm and falls short of the wrist and they get paraesthesia in the hands... The ECG can be normal but what the patient tells you can be important; I try to get that across to the students.'

The expert was comparing this patient's symptoms with a typical scenario. In addition, she was building a case to support her diagnosis by identifying underpinning physiological changes. She drew on her experience of similar cases and compared them with the symptoms this patient was exhibiting. In addition, she had sufficient knowledge to know that the patient's experience could be more informative in diagnosis setting than an ECG reading.

Specialists' knowledge

In the main, specialists had distinctive roles such as breast care nurses, stoma therapists, Macmillan nurses, TPN (total parenteral nutrition) advisors and control of infection nurses. They were aware of their own distinctive knowledge and were used as consultants by ward and community based nurses. They had three subdivisions, which had similarities to (a) the Humanistic Existentialist group (b) the Traditionalist group and (c) the Technologist group. While they had similarities with each of the other groups, they also shared characteristics among themselves which ensured their distinctiveness as a group.

Specialists demonstrated a wide range of knowledge. For example, some prescribed and recommended medication. They had knowledge of anatomy and physiology and disease processes. They had the knowledge to carry out assessments. They also synthesised subject matter knowledge and experience to give nursing care. They demonstrated a diagnostic ability and they were able to assess patients' quality of life and evaluate possible actions in the light of this. They had the knowledge to make certain situations transformative in that they were able to go beyond the superficial and establish underlying causes for concern or for specific action. They had all developed distinct specialist knowledge in terms of the speciality in which they worked. Well-developed communication and counselling abilities were displayed and many of these nurses had extended their practice into what was previously the doctor's territory. One nurse, for example, was inserting central venous pressure (CVP) lines successfully and another was administering chemotherapy.

Specialists identified complications of disease processes and medication. This ability may not in itself be considered an advanced form of nursing care; a relatively junior nurse might well be aware that morphine can cause constipation. Rather, their expertise was evident in that they not only remembered the various complications that might arise (when others did not) but they were alerted to a possible diagnosis even when presented with apparently contradictory evidence. This identification ability is evident in the following example given by a Macmillan nurse:

'I can think of a lady who had been on the books for some time and she had been fairly stable. She was a breast, ...I think she had received chemotherapy and radiotherapy and was getting on with living her life. We were going in intermittently at this stage because she was not needing active contact. The daughter rang and said that her Mom had been acting a bit funny. We asked what she meant and she explained that her Mom seemed a bit vacant at times. The patient was only in her 40s; you would not expect her to be behaving in the way that she was.

We went in to have a chat and see what was happening and found that the doctor had been in the previous week and had given her some [anti] emetics because she was being intermittently sick. We watched her walking and her gait was altered; it was fairly obvious to us that there was more going on there than just an associated nausea. So we had to go back to the doctor and report these other things that were going on and the doctor said right away that perhaps we ought to get her scanned. He had not picked up the other things in the first place.

Caudal pressure is the other one that we get hot under the collar about and is often missed. You often get the situation of wide-spread bone mets. [metastasis] especially with the prostrate and the breast — they tend to pick up a lot of widespread bone mets, and you get someone who is starting to say that they have got pins and needles, sensory loss or numbness or they can't walk properly or their foot keeps going cold that to us is a sign that something is going on that we need to do something about, but other professionals tend to sit on that. Like the problems of constipation in the terminally ill. It is there to the fore of your mind — is there something else going on?

If this lady's daughter had not had contact with us as a specialist team then those symptoms would not have been picked up until much later. Her mother did have some radiotherapy and she was put on dexamethasone, and she did continue to have some quality of life.'

Clearly, this nurse was able to recognise early warning signals that all was not well with the patient. Less experienced nurses might wait to receive further cues before progressing with any further investigations. Expertise is demonstrated in the early detection of worrying symptoms and the ability to make tentative judgements based on limited information.

In terms of giving advice to doctors, an expert nurse who works in terminal care explained how vulnerable she feels:

'I think in the present situation I feel vulnerable when ...[doctors ask advice about methods of treatment] ... we have all been brought up on the old school of you will do, you will not do, and those restrictions, and of course we are in to legal worries now.'

These factors concerned the expert nurse considerably.

'I do get quite alarmed with the situation that is happening sometimes... where the consultant will say to the houseman, talk to X, she will tell you what to do. It is nice in one way but it is an awful responsibility and it is a responsibility I am very aware of. I wasn't in clinic the other day [and] a different decision was made on a protocol that had been pre-worked out, ...[the] consultant, junior doctor and myself have sat down and worked out a protocol of treatment and a wrong decision was made and a patient was sent for chemotherapy when he had a squamous cell and he should not have had chemotherapy. I had a phone call on the Monday morning from the junior doctor to say "I did this on Wednesday, was that right?" I said "Well, usually it would have been radiotherapy" and the treatment was cancelled, just on my say so, just like that they cancelled his chemotherapy and sent him for radiotherapy. Now I think that is an awesome responsibility. It is the consultant's responsibility but at the end of the day the practicality was that the junior doctor rang me.'

This nurse clearly conveys the sense of responsibility that she felt in this situation. She was prepared to advise the junior doctor as to what was usual in terms of treatment for a patient with this type of condition, but giving this information was not easy. Indeed, she perceived this as an awesome responsibility. Such concerns are not linked with issues of knowledge or lack of it, for the expert nurse was party to the writing of a protocol for patient management. Rather, what is significant is that the nurse was concerned about the consequences of her actions. The consequence of this nurse giving the doctor information was that a patient's treatment was changed. It is likely that this nurse's concerns are linked to the fact that, traditionally, nurses acted as assistants to and for doctors. While such nurses extended their knowledge bases, they were nonetheless in a sense secure because doctors accepted responsibility for their suggestions. With the increasing proactivity and autonomy being undertaken by specialist nurses however, this security has gone. These are issues that they are having to learn to address.

Quality of life

Consideration and estimation of patients' quality of life were significant features in the knowledge bases held by specialist nurses. In discussion with an expert stoma therapist, it emerged that being able to judge a patient's quality of life was an essential part of her knowledge base:

> 'If I already know the patient then obviously I have an assessment already of that patient's capabilities, whether they are going to be able to cope with a long term problem, or whether they are going to fold and say "I can't cope with this any more", in that case the quality of life ...we have got to sort out for this patient, if it is going to be that bad, then it's worth the risk of surgery, even if it would not be ideal.

If the patient of eighty plus has a temporary stoma for acute obstruction and then four months later comes the day when the surgeon says "Well look I don't really want to put this back for you, it is going to be difficult, blah, blah, blah" and I know the patient is sort of saying "I hate this, I hate this" that to me says look OK, the patient knows all the odds, they know they might have problems, they know they might not come through the operation but it is worth the risk because of the quality of life.'

In this example, the expert nurse recognises that in certain circumstances what may appear to be an unacceptable risk to a surgeon may be perceived differently by the patient. For example, a patient whose quality of life is very poor and who has great difficulty in coming to terms with a stoma may decide that s/he is prepared to accept the risks of additional surgery.

Transformative ability

The ability to listen to what the patient or relatives are saying and to transform a difficult situation into a manageable one is demonstrated in the following example given by an expert Macmillan nurse:

'A GP was unhappy. He kept getting called out to a terminally ill patient, for what he considered to be trivial reasons, eg. the relatives were calling him out and saying things like "Mom's got a nasty taste in her mouth" or "She keeps getting cramp in her legs". I asked the GP if he felt the relatives wanted to talk through what was happening with their mother. His response was that "They know that she is dying". My feelings were that, yes, they might know that she was dying but they may not be able to express their feelings about that and they may not fully understand what the process is going to be and they might need more information as to how to handle the situation...'

Consequently, the expert nurse visited the family and asked:

> 'Did they understand what was happening and were there things they wanted to ask about and it went on from there. ... He [the doctor] made the comment that it had been "A lot quieter since you have been going in"... He did recognise that the trivial visits were a cry for help but he did not know how to handle them. Once the patient and family were able to express their feelings, the trivial visits did stop.'

In this example, the nurse had the knowledge to recognise that the so-called trivial visits were a cry for help. Although the relatives knew that their mother was going to die, they did not know what this process might involve and needed reassurance. The expert nurse recognised that there was a difference between being aware that a relative was dying and understanding what that process might involve. It seemed as if the doctor in this instance saw acceptance that a relative is going to die as being synonymous with understanding the process. It is apparent that in close nurse-patient relationships, the nurse is able to view the situation from the relatives' perspective rather than from a distanced professional perspective. Life experience is likely to be influential in enabling nurses to perceive relatives or patients as 'another self' (Orem, 1980).

Challenging medical staff

One specialist wondered if having the ability to challenge medical staff was a characteristic of being an expert nurse. She asked:

> 'Do you think the expert nurse is the one who has stood up to medical staff and is prepared to say "I don't agree with this". Even when I was a casualty sister, the medical staff would say, "This patient could go home" and if I was concerned I would say "Are you sure?" and we would have

this big discussion and I would say my bit and he would say his, and I would say "Well, I am keeping the patient in anyway" and I would keep him all night and do observations all night and the first time in the morning that he peed, and it was all full of blood, I would say, "There, told you so!" Perhaps the people who are able to stick their neck out have always been able to stick their neck out.'

Analysis of the data (Conway, 1995) reveals several experts who identified that, in the past, they were always in some sense different; they were prepared to intervene on their patient's behalf regardless of how junior they were. However, there was not any direct linkage between personality or motivation and expertise. Some experts came into nursing in order to have a job, whereas others viewed it as a vocation. In addition, while some were assertive others were not.

Traditionalists' knowledge

Traditionalists operated very much along 'traditional ward sister lines'. They monitored the actions of patients and nurses. They were generally lacking in awareness of their own worth and seemed surprised by the amount and type of knowledge that they used in their own nursing practice. As one expert stated:

'I don't think we realise how much we do do.'

A medical model guided their practice. It was as if these experts had a range of possibilities in terms of what was acceptable for a given medical condition in their heads. They constantly monitored to ensure that patients were not falling outside of these parameters.

Experience strongly influenced their actions. There was scant evidence of theoretical frameworks being used to guide care provision. Managerial responsibility was a major factor for these nurses. They were all either sister grade or directorate nurse grade. Their expertise seemed to have developed in terms of survival. They were mainly preoccupied with 'getting the work done' and managing care with scarce resources. They operated very much as overseers and assistants to doctors. Also, they had learnt how to keep patients' complaints to a minimum. They believed that they had little or no management support.

Field notes from one of the observation visits contained these impressions following a visit to an expert nurse from this group.

> 'General impressions rather mixed, ...appeared quite old fashioned in many respects, ie. needed to keep an eye on everything herself, very friendly and helpful to both staff and patients. Sat in on a report where there were huge number of patients to be reported on. Lot of time spent getting to know all of the patients, almost all of the morning. Seemed to feel she had to check up and keep an eye on staff. Much of the care given on ward seemed to be routinised. Doctors seemed to come before patients, ie. expert gave attention to medical staff when a patient also needed attention. Knowledge base seemed to be related to medical, physical aspects of care (although in-depth knowledge not so obviously identifiable). Concerned to know everything. Lack of appreciation of staff. Lack of appreciation of nursing role, seems to be perceived not so much as a therapeutic process, rather as a job needing doing. Staff not actively encouraged to accept responsibility, sister still mopped up. Emphasis on petty things, eg. staff were not allowed to use new envelopes, had to tell staff nurse to put letter in an envelope, had to find the new envelope for the staff nurse. Lack of perception of ability to change or alter things. Little or no evidence of challenging. Nursing viewed from nurses' perspective rather than patients' perspective.'

These general impressions were arrived at from observation of the expert nurse in practice. Resources, or lack of them, feature prominently in these nurses' agendas and they presented themselves as powerless as a result of NHS reforms. They were concerned with trying to maintain standards but were aware that they were unable to do this in a time of cost containment. It was as if these nurses were under siege both from management and at times from doctors, and they were concerned to protect their staff. An expert from a medical area endeavoured to ensure that actions carried out by nurses did not leave them open to criticism, censure or legal action.

These experts displayed a monitoring function which focused on the nursing staff, in terms of correcting them rather than correcting the doctors. There was also a monitoring role in respect of protecting junior staff from what the medical staff might ask them to do. Although these experts identified that they could be assertive on occasions, they were largely non-assertive and reactive when dealing with doctors. While the technologist group had extended their knowledge well into the province of doctors' knowledge, this was not apparent with this group.

Monitoring

During a visit to a vascular-surgery ward, an expert nurse was observed carrying out many monitoring functions. She checked notes and X-rays to make sure that they were complete and available and she also ensured that any problems in pathological reports were dealt with. The expert explained that she was looking for things like prothrombin times (to monitor that it was safe for the patient to undergo surgery):

'When the consultants are ready to do the round, I check that the X-rays are there, especially reports on barium enemas. There is one lady who has had one done at lunch time [barium enema] that won't be reported on ...I will make a note this evening for the ward clerk to go and fetch the report first thing in the morning. There is a chance that the patient might be able to go home if we get the report.'

She was observed waiting on various doctors, fetching and carrying for them and generally making life easier for them. She presented this role very much as a monitoring one, in that she ensured that situations which concerned her were brought to the doctor's attention. She explained her thinking in relation to medical rounds:

'Make sure patients are on their beds, make sure the treatment cards are there. I feel doing the round is our time for bringing out what the patients are feeling, because the patients won't tell the doctor. Mary would never have mentioned her back pain to Mr M... [the surgeon]. I think it is our time to be the patient's advocate.'

This expert nurse was observed fetching patients notes from the office for the doctor. When asked why she did this, she explained that:

'I thought in the back of my mind that the doctor could get on with examining the patient if I went and got the notes.'

She was also observed telling the doctor the patient's diagnosis as he came to each patient. When asked why she did this, she replied:

'I don't think he can remember all the patients and sometimes he just needs a little refresher.'

From these examples, it is evident that the expert nurse viewed the doctor's time as more important than her own, and that she was prepared to assume a subservient role so that she could ensure the patients she felt needed seeing were, in fact, seen by a doctor.

The expert also carried out a monitoring function in relation to the patient's notes. The expert nurse identified that:

> 'Mrs A came in; she was for vascular surgery and she had some bloods checked and her INR [prothrombin level] was 3.3 which is high. We stopped her Warfarin, but we still needed to have a check to make sure it was within normal levels before she went to theatre and this was the test that she had, which was more acceptable. It is a little bit on the slow side if anything, the control was 35 and hers was 31 secs... It is the ratio that is important if it is anything over 40, the one lady we had hers was 165, in which case I immediately stopped the Heparin and told the doctors. Often the doctors have asked for these, but they might never see the result, so we do put them out for them to see. If there was something really abnormal I would put them out for them to see. I also look for things like patients' Hbs, high ureas, glucose levels.'

This monitoring and action-initiating role, in relation to pathological reports, has received scant attention in the nursing literature. The expert nurse felt it was an important aspect of her role but it appears to be an aspect that is not formally acknowledged. The expert nurse also appeared to be establishing priorities:

> 'I wanted to find out for my own peace of mind, I'm sure that if a staff nurse had been in charge that she would have also wanted to check that problems are not going to arise later on, especially [after] five o'clock [when] the doctors go...'

These experts at times displayed a maternal role both towards their nursing staff and to the doctors. They saw themselves as having the knowledge to be supportive to junior staff who were dealing with emotionally draining situations.

> 'Sometimes situations can be very depressing, particularly with terminally ill patients, especially with junior staff but it can be quite satisfying too, even though it is a very sad occasion, to console relatives and make them feel better. This is something positive that can be done in a negative situation.'

One expert recounted how she tried to draw on her previous knowledge of patient care situations so that she could recount positive examples, such as talking about patients who you never ever thought would pull through and of how, against the odds, they made it. She felt that this knowledge from experience enabled her to provide an alternative perspective to more junior staff, who could be overwhelmed when caring for people with terminal illness.

Acting as an interpreter

Interpreting is seen as important by these experts. This was clearly demonstrated by one expert immediately following a ward round. She returned to a patient who had been told that she could go home by the doctor, to check that the patient had fully understood what the doctor had said. This expert nurse explained:

> 'Sometimes especially with a foreign doctor, they talk and the patient does not understand.'

This interpreting role was concerned with much more than language difference; it seemed to be concerned with establishing the reality of the patient's comprehension in relation to what the doctor had been saying. This involved 'interpreting' medical jargon into a form that the patient could understand.

Powerlessness

These experts seemed largely reactive to change and appeared to have few strategies for dealing with the change process apart from endeavouring as far as possible, and within the resources available, to struggle to maintain standards. This lack of ability to bring about change was demonstrated by an expert who expressed a sense of 'helplessness' in terms of the cross-infection that was occurring in her ward area:

> 'Every child we have coming back from ... hospital following surgery, or because they have been referred to us because we are the local hospital, always has rota-virus. This goes around the ward like wild fire. We have found that children are coming in for one complaint, being admitted to us and then contracting a rota-virus here, so after they are discharged for say bronchiolitis, they are then admitted with diarrhoea. We have had control of infection lectures here and we have had the ward washed down, but there is still a feeling that we are giving children rota-virus. Going back a few years to when I did my training, if there was an infectious child in a cubicle, when they went home the cubicle was washed down or fumigated, but nothing like that happens now, so at half past eight in the morning you can have a child with rota-virus and they may be discharged and the bed and locker and everything else is washed down and the linen is changed and say about ten o'clock at night you get another child admitted to that cubicle, because of pressure on cubicles, and you can almost guarantee that that child will pick up rota-virus, even though we are quite strict on isolation techniques.'

Several factors appear influential in the development of expertise in the traditionalist group. An expert from a children's ward explained that:

'I think my expertise just happened rather than being taught. I had to learn as I went along.'

Practice had been significant for this expert in terms of developing her expertise. She described the influence of the socialisation process on her when she was a student:

'When I started my training, the sisters were the experts and I used to think that the staff nurses were little gods. I saw them as different to the sisters of today. Sisters were very professional and you don't get that to the same extent today... I can remember Sr Lewis on the medical ward dishing out the meals which some might say is a waste of time, but when you went for the meal with your tray, she would say, "Nurse, what food values are in this meal?" so she was teaching and acting as a role model all the time. This sort of approach made me want to be the best also.'

The importance of early role models is evident in this example, where the expert nurse identifies her feelings of admiration and expresses a desire to emulate those sisters from her training days:

'The students do not look upon me with the same respect, well I don't think they do any sister. If, when I was a student, you were in the office and a sister came in, you would automatically stand up and you would go out or go and do something else. If you were with the sister in the office and a nursing officer came in you would automatically say excuse me and go out. They don't today; they just stand there and you have to say, "Would you mind leaving the office". I think a bit of the professionalism has gone. They [traditional ward sisters] were a bit hierarchical I suppose, but they really had got the patient's welfare at heart.'

Clearly apparent within this statement is a sense of nostalgia for traditional values and a sense that ways of behaving in the past were better.

Professionalism in this statement is synonymous with outward signs of behaviour or etiquette, such as standing up when a senior nurse came into the office.

Monitoring staff

During an observation visit to another expert from a medical area, it was evident that she saw herself as needing to check up and monitor her staff:

Interviewer: ' ...[why did you tell] a staff nurse who was drawing up some insulin to take the insulin with him?'

Expert: 'Because I noted that when he drew up the insulin he checked it with the other staff nurse, but he put the vial back in the fridge, so I asked him to take the insulin [vial] with him.'

Interviewer: 'Because?'

Expert: 'Well because obviously, obvious to me but it was not obvious to him, ... if he had to put that down, nobody would know what was in it. I find sometimes that the male nurses tend to do things for convenience. Maybe I am being biased there, but we have had a few problems in that way just recently. I have had more than my fair share of male nurses and maybe, that is why we are noticing it more. Sometimes they seem to do things for the easy way out, not necessarily negligent in their fashion, but it could be negligent if something happened and they tend to sort of think, "If I get rid of that now, I have not got to put it away afterwards and if I have locked the fridge I have not got to open it again to put the thing away". That kind of thing and that was what I was trying to get at really. He needed to make sure that he knew what was in, and everybody else knew what was in, that syringe.'

It is clearly demonstrated in this incident that the expert nurse felt that she had a strong teaching and monitoring role in relation to this staff nurse. She had strong views about how a procedure should be carried out and felt that to carry it out any other way was unsafe and poor practice. The expert nurse believed that not only did the staff nurse have to do things properly, but that it was necessary for him to do this in such a way that others would know what he was doing. Also evident is the fact that the expert nurse did not appear to accept that the staff nurse was accountable for his own practice, rather than merely doing as he was told. The expert then pointed out to the staff nurse that he should give the auxiliary he was working with a report. The expert was asked:

> **Interviewer:** *'Would he not have done that without you pointing it out?'*

> **Expert:** *'He may have done and he may not have done, well, he has not been on here himself long and he is still feeling his way as it were. He came from an ITU situation and to slip from an ITU to a ward like this, well it is very different and he has not found it very easy to slip back into that role of sort of general nurse, and he thinks sort of technical, you know. I won't say that he does not look at the patient holistically... He does not look at it in the way we do in a general ward area. He was probably one of the most junior staff in the ITU, whereas here he is one of the most senior... He tends sometimes to be not aware of the fact or aware of how little his juniors understand or know.'*

There are several important issues in this transcript. The expert nurse clearly felt that this staff nurse was not yet looking at things 'in the way we do in a general ward area'. It seemed that she accepted, apparently unquestioningly, the fact that this staff nurse was very junior in an ITU situation, but she did not find it inappropriate that this quite junior nurse should now accept considerable responsibility (albeit heavily monitored) on an acute medical ward, where he was perceived as 'one of the most senior'. It further became apparent that this sister was dissatisfied with many of the activities of the nursing staff in her absence. A used instrument tray with bloodstained instruments had been left in a side area:

> 'Which [I] intend to take up with Heather [staff nurse] afterwards ...she was the one who told me it had been there two days. They [the nurses] are trying to indoctrinate the doctors these days with the attitude, you must get rid of your sharps, obviously because of risks with hepatitis, etc and the doctor knows where he has used the sharps, well that is fair comment, but there were no needles there, or used syringes there, the equipment has obviously got to go to HSDU [Hospital Sterilising Disinfectant Unit] and should have been cleared away... Some doctors do of course, I mean they clear everything away, but knowing Dr X as well as I do, I know darn well he is not going to clear a trolley away, it is all you can do to get him to write a prescription form' (chuckle).

There are several significant points in this transcript. The expert once again feels that she needs to reprimand a member of her staff. She understands that the nursing staff are trying to encourage the doctors to clear away the instruments they have used, but felt that one of the nursing staff should have assumed responsibility for clearing the tray away. Most telling is the fact that she accepts that Dr X not only would not clear a trolley away, but also 'it is all you can do to get him to write a prescription form'. This comment was followed by a wry chuckle which seemed to indicate a type of indulgence towards this doctor, almost as if she accepts he is behaving in an unreasonable way but is prepared to accept this because of who he is.

The expert nurse interpreted views which were different from hers as suspect in origin. A staff nurse suggested that a patient who had experienced a sub-arachnoid haemorrhage should be catheterised:

> 'I can't see his logic there. She had been incontinent during the night, well that is fair comment. The lady has had a sub-arachnoid haemorrhage and she probably went off into a deep sleep. To me, well to anybody really, I would think it is an excuse for catheterisation if somebody is incontinent. I think that is just an excuse for keeping a dry bed.'

Clearly the expert perceives herself as having the patient's best welfare at heart, a fact that she does not feel is shared by all of the nursing staff. The expert was keen to ensure that patients were cared for correctly and that she was aware of everything that needed doing. She revealed that the relatives of one patient had complained about the care their mother had received, so when she heard that this patient's naso-gastric tube had been removed she was quite concerned.

> 'I am a bit concerned. My concern is not as real as you would expect here, I just wanted to clarify that they [the nursing staff] had made a sort of a sensible decision about this lady, because we have had problems, not with her, because she is a sweet little soul but certainly with her family from the beginning.'

The expert nurse was trying to establish areas that might potentially be contentious in the future. She was also trying to ensure that complaints were minimalised and that nursing staff did things 'properly' and did not leave themselves open to censure. The expert's primary response seemed to be to smooth the situation over and the daughter was perceived as over-protective.

> 'I spent probably about four hours with that family because they were so concerned, in fact the daughter is over-protective, ...she wanted her observed every minute.'

While maintenance of standards was presented as important to these expert nurses such standards arose from the 'world view' held by these experts. An expert from a children's ward explained that she had her own standards and that there were certain activities that she felt had to be carried out in a particular manner.

> 'There are certain things on the ward that I am a stickler for, for example temperature charts. I don't see the need for a constipation to have his temperature done everyday the same with the lodger. I don't see why we should do a temperature, if the child has not got a temperature, but there again, if a child has got a temperature, then I expect the chart to be completed and I don't mean just ticks.
>
> If a child has had his bowels open I expect a description of the stool, if they are a diarrhoea. If children are on a temperature chart, then I want a respiratory rate done, because I know that the consultants especially with the asthmatic children and the pneumonias, look at the respiratory rate and as the temperature comes down, the respiratory rate usually comes down also.'

The importance of other members of staff carrying out nursing duties to the standard set by the expert nurse is clearly evidenced here. This expert placed considerable emphasis on tasks being carried out in a prescribed way. Also apparent was the depersonalised way children were referred to as conditions, that is, a child is a constipation, or a lodger, or diarrhoea. This reflects an approach to care which is heavily influenced by a medical diagnosis, and where the patient is viewed almost as the doctor's property. Activities are primarily being carried out because the consultant will want to know. There is an absence of any recognition that other members of the nursing staff are autonomous practitioners in their own right.

Humanistic Existentialists' knowledge

These experts used a strong nursing focus for care provision. Also, a philosophy of humanism permeated their practice. Subject matter knowledge was complex. Their practice was underpinned with theories from the social sciences and nursing. Their practice was an amalgam of theoretical knowledge, values, experience and subject matter knowledge. Their knowledge enabled them to be pro-active in terms of their practice. They also demonstrated strong ownership of the knowledge they used and developed. These experts integrated theories into practice thus linking the theory-practice gap. Reflection and reflective abilities were the hallmark of the Humanistic Existentialists. They demonstrated critical awareness about themselves and others. They contributed to a nurturing environment which acted like a breeding ground for expertise development.

Artistry was evident in their practice. This included a phenomenological ability where they were able to enter into the 'real world' of the patient and see things from the patient's view point. Poetry, aromatherapy and meditation were used by some to provide holistic care. They also exhibited a transformative ability where apparently intractable problems were turned into positive situations.

Artistry in nursing

Earlier scenarios reflect knowledge use in terms of the scientific and technical aspects of nursing. However, expert nursing also has an art side to it. Humanistic experts and, to a lesser extent, some of the other experts demonstrated the ability to get into the 'real world' of the clients they were caring for. This is described as phenomenology-in-action.

Phenomenology-in-action

The following example illustrates an almost instantaneous assessment process carried out by an expert surgical nurse:

'When I am introduced to a client, or to take over their care... or whatever, I am not that interested in the details. I go straight for the patient and I go over to [them] and [ask] how are you and whatever, I go straight into that, regardless of you know, endless information that the nurse wants to tell me about what she has done and the temperature is this, and the urine output is that, the drains are this, I just go straight to the patient.'

In this extract the expert nurse identified the ability she had to go directly to a patient and to make judgements about that patient's care. She was sufficiently secure in her knowledge base to accept the 'world as presented by the patient' as a basis for her judgements. She explained that she was not particularly concerned with the patient's diagnosis at this stage:

'I pick that up, I don't worry about that, in looking at them and assessing them, from an observational point of view, if they are fit enough to engage in conversation with me, I get a real sense of where they are, I get a sense of whether they are unstable or not and then I prioritise accordingly, but I can go straight for the patient. I think that is where I am different. I am beginning to make sense of their world.'

This beginning to make sense of a patient's world is an intriguing concept.

Interviewer: *'In other words you are establishing a shared world with them?'*

Expert: *'I engage with them straight away and that is a very rapid assessment, it is almost, well it is almost* *instantaneous, although it isn't because, obviously, there is some cognition and everything else going on [laughter]. But it is pretty quick, and I know that staff nurses who hand over to me can feel very uncertain of that approach... they will be looking for external observable parameters, how much urine, how many days post op, are we in to more fluids yet, what is the pain, how much do they know about the diagnosis. They are not really going through a checklist but, depending on how senior they are, they are doing clusters of care, they are perhaps thinking about the physical care issues, they are still separating psychological issues, whereas I don't think I do, I think I just take it as the patient presents it. And I will work with that, so it is my inter-personal skills and my ability to assess I think [that] are quite sophisticated and then that is supported obviously by a relevant knowledge base, and I can make sense of those observations very, very quickly. I think the other thing is, that from that, I get a very clear sense of priority of care... What are the important things that have to be dealt with, what are important but can be left for a while?... I think patients recognise being cared for by me is different ... it is something else, a combination of those things when they all come together. There is something extra as well that they recognise, that they are safe in my hands, that may or may not be true [laughs] but they perceive something about my demeanour and my approach, and that is why I work in that particular way. It gives them a sense of safety, that I know what I am on about, that they are safe in my care.'*

Here the expert nurse demonstrated clear analytical ability in relation to her practice. She compared and contrasted her practice with that of less experienced nurses, and devised explanations for the differences in the way assessment was carried out by her. She demonstrated reflective ability in terms of how she presented to patients, and she deconstructed the processes she used, so that she was able to provide a rationale for her approach. In terms of the process of entering a patient world the interviewer asked:

Interviewer: *'Are you conscious of what if anything you are thinking about...?'*

Expert: *' I have got a kind of set in my mind of what I might expect an individual going through this experience to be at. What stage they might be at. So I am doing a kind of matching process, I mean I have got fifteen years of surgical nursing and I have come across most situations many, many times, so I have a kind of internal picture of what some one four days post-op should be about. It is not necessarily terribly scientific or anything you know rigid, it is quite flexible, but it is nonetheless there, so I think when I am going in on a first encounter I have got that mental set that I refer to.*

I mean I am quite comfortable when people are out of that set and I can work out why, but it is when they don't fit and there is no reason why they don't fit, then my ears and whiskers are up and I am searching harder, and then I start to become more methodical to ensure that I have not missed something...

There are times when I catch myself out, I get a sense of "this isn't right" and then I haven't actually necessarily got a sense of the full details of the operation. I go back to the operating notes and find, well, they [the patient] have not got a colon so no wonder they have got this, or whatever it is, and I have made an assumption somewhere along the line... so I have to go back and clarify in order to assure myself why someone is out of the "set" and secure a rationale for it.'

Interviewer: *'If a nurse was handing over to you and giving you a report on a patient, how much information do you actually want from her?'*

Expert: *'I like to know the name of the patient... if we are at the bedside and she is telling me about what she has* *done all morning, I am not interested. I am sitting there observing the patient, I am making almost my own assessment in defiance of the information she is very keen to tell me. I notice that the more senior, more experienced nurses start to move along the way I do in that they will just give you the essence of the morning and I look at some of the handovers between relatively junior staff and it is probably quite appropriate that it is a list of things and then that person makes sense of their own list of things because that is the way that they operate and that is the way they get their confidence to handle the situation.'*

The explanations about patient assessment were clearly presented and followed both a deductive and a reflection-in-action model (Schon, 1987). The expert nurse showed that she came to an interaction with an open mind informed by a mental set based on expectations of patients' conditions and responses. This had been built up over fifteen years of practice, and was informed by a knowledge base derived from both nursing and social sciences. She was able through a process of observation to make a very rapid assessment of the patient's condition. She quickly detected if the patient was not conforming to the mental set she used for assessment. The confidence the expert had in her judgmental ability was clearly illustrated in the transcript.

She was single-minded in terms of establishing priorities and planning patient care, trusted her own judgement and was rather impatient of well-meaning but, to the expert, irrelevant explanations about care that had been given. There is an interesting line where the expert said 'I am making almost my own assessment in defiance of the information she is very keen to tell me'. The nurse in this sentence seemed to be saying that she knew that looking at and talking to the patient would tell her more than any hand-over from the staff nurse could have done.

Her use of the word 'defiance' is indicative of the expert rejecting a rational, explicit approach to care (or at least suspending it) in favour of an approach which has more in common with the art side of nursing and is akin to an intuitive process. Although this is not a scientific process, from her explanation it is clear that her actions had some elements of reflection-in-action and of knowing-in-action in them (Schon, 1987).

This phenomenological approach has several important characteristics. First, the expert approaches the patient with an open mind. Secondly, a process of matching takes place. At this stage the expert nurse is drawing on not only theoretical, formal knowledge, for example psychology, physiology, disease processes, but also on experiential knowledge which includes mental sets of a range of 'normal scenarios'. Thirdly, the expert nurse is able to detect when some of the cues do not match a normal range of scenarios and she is then able to obtain further information to establish the significance of these cues. The expert recognises that her approach gives her a degree of credibility with her patients.

This ability was also demonstrated by experts from other groups so does not seem to be the sole province of the Humanistic Existentialists. However, the humanistic experts were the only group to demonstrate insight and awareness of this process. An example of this ability was demonstrated by an expert Traditionalist nurse from a medical area during an observation visit. The expert was talking to a patient in a side ward. The patient had been quite ill and was finding it difficult to eat an adequate diet and build up her strength. The expert lapsed into the same local dialect as the patient and her accent became very pronounced during the interaction. It was as if the expert nurse was saying through the use of the accent 'you and I are of the same stock, therefore I understand you, and you understand me and this is a strength in our relationship'. The expert spoke bluntly to the patient outlining her options. The expert was asked why she had handled the interaction in the way she had. She explained:

'I felt there was no point in waffling around with this little lady because that was what she understood, I don't know why I was like that with her. It just seemed to be the right way with her.'

In this example the expert demonstrated the ability to enter into the same world as the patient. This appeared to be an intuitive process where the expert nurse knew that it was appropriate to talk to the patient in a very matter-of-fact way and to use an accent almost as broad as the patient's. She saw this as a way of gaining credibility with the patient.

Artistry in practice

Artistry can present in many forms, for example, as therapeutic interventions and through the use of complementary therapies, such as massage, aromatherapy and meditation. In the following excerpt, an expert Humanistic Existentialist explained how she integrated poetry into her nursing practice:

'One of the important things that I use in my work is poetry,... and Yeats is probably my favourite poet. ...You know you work through things like the Ode to a Nightingale by Keats, sort of when he describes the dying process. I can't remember the exact words but [he] talks about sailing into Bysantium and that is about old age isn't it?'

She also used music when caring for patients.

'I have just got some money to buy a Walkman for our own team, to allow people to listen to music. I use it to give therapy.'

For this expert, nursing is about much more than just carrying out tasks. It is about caring for the whole person.

This involves not only operating from a scientific basis but also utilisation of the art side of nursing as well.

She described an incident where she had been caring for an elderly woman who was diagnosed as having cancer of the uterus. The expert presented the patient as having Victorian values. The son and daughter were very caring and visited frequently. They did not want their mother to be told her diagnosis. The expert described how a close and deep relationship developed between herself and this elderly woman who subsequently asked her if she had in fact got cancer.

Knowing the wishes of the family, the expert nurse was at first evasive and attempted to contact the patient's daughter, so that she could ask her to come to the hospital as she felt the patient should be told. The expert in the event did tell the patient and the relatives accepted this, but following this disclosure, the patient refused to talk to her family and communicated only at a superficial level with the nurse. This continued for five to six days and the patient seemed more and more withdrawn. This concerned the expert as she felt she had been instrumental in bringing this about. A colleague suggested that the patient was, in fact, demonstrating the stages of grief as described by Kubler Ross (1973).

Although this provided an explanation, it did not alter the situation, and the family and the nurse were feeling excluded. A nursing colleague had the idea of using the ward's pictorial philosophy to 'get through' to the patient:

'...we did not have a [written] ward philosophy stuck on the ward, we had a pictorial philosophy which was a lovely idea. The philosophy was in the front and there was all photographs of patients all the way through and a little bit of the philosophy was put under each page as appropriate and it shows nurses and patients together, interacting.'

The expert took the philosophy to the patient:

> '..."can I leave this on your table, you might want to look at it?" Don't ask me why, but I had a "gut feeling" that if I left it there and left it open, that she may look at it. I went back a couple of hours later ...and she looked ...and then she said "This book here ...it is good isn't it?" I said "in what way?" and she said "I did not know that nurses sat down and wrote philosophies like this ...I knew they cared, but I did not know that they really thought about it, these photographs ...look at that nurse especially, she really, really cares"...'

As this elderly woman's life drew to a close, above all else she really wanted to go home and sit in her garden. The expert nurse set about arranging this. Permission was obtained and the nurse called to take the patient home. Unfortunately, the patient now felt too weak to cope with the journey so the visit had to be cancelled. Arrangements had been made for one of the doctors who was off duty at five o'clock to call and take tea with the patient, the nurses and her daughter, but this all had to be cancelled.

> 'I spoke to the daughter and I said "[if] we can't take her to the garden can [we] not bring the garden to her?" '

This was exactly what the daughter and the expert nurse did. They ensured that the patient's side ward was transformed into a garden.

> 'In the event lots and lots of flowers were brought in from the garden, tulips and daffodils. They were absolutely glorious.'

The tea party was now carried out in the patient's room with her daughter, nurse and doctor present. The patient died four days later.

Perhaps this nurse did not have to be an expert to carry out the actions she did. She did, however, need a nursing focus to care so that she saw the patient as an individual with needs. This nurse needed to think creatively and imaginatively so that she could help the patient to have some pleasure in her last days. The expert also needed knowledge of the patient's condition so that she was able to present realistic possibilities to the patient. Caring and openness are evident in this example.

Conclusion

Any discussion about nursing expertise needs to recognise the intuitive art side of nursing. While 'gut feelings' and caring cannot be scientifically quantified they can and do make a significant difference to the care-giving process. It can be seen that the development of appropriate attitudes and values is as important to developing expertise in nursing as gaining knowledge about carrying out tasks or undertaking a particular form of study.

References

Benner P (1984) *From Novice to Expert: Excellence and Power in Clinical Practice*. Addison-Wesley, California

Carper BA (1978) Fundamental patterns of knowing in nursing. *Adv Nurs Sci* **1**(1): 13–23

Conway J (1995) *Expert Nursing Knowledge as an Evolutionary Process*. Unpublished PhD Thesis, University of Warwick, Coventry

Fitzpatrick J, While AE, Roberts JD (1992) The role of the nurse in high-quality patient care: a review of the literature. *J Adv Nurs* **17**: 1210–9

Hyland T (1993) Professional development and competence-based education. *Educ Stud* **19**(1): 123–32

Kubler-Ross E (1973) *On Death and Dying*. Tavistock Publications, London

McCaugherty D (1992a) The gap between nursing theory and practice. *Sen Nurse* **12**(6): 44–8

McCaugherty D (1992b) The concepts of theory and practice. *Sen Nurse* **30**(122): 29–33

Orem DE (1980) *Nursing Concepts of Practice*. McGraw Hill, New York

Schon DA (1983) *The Reflective Practitioner: How Professionals Think in Action*. Basic Books Inc, New York

Schon DA (1987) *Educating the Reflective Practitioner*. Jossey-Bass, London

Chapter 6

Cultural influences on knowledge development and expertise

Advancing practice and developing expertise is about much more than taking on additional tasks or attending a specialised course. The culture that nurses work in, and their relationship to that culture, is a highly significant factor in this process. This chapter explores cultural influences and relationships in terms of advancing practice and developing expertise.

Culture is defined in a number of ways, for example as 'the customs and civilisation of a particular people or group' (Oxford Paperback Dictionary). It has links with the socialisation process (Collins New World Thesaurus). The word culture is used here in the context of the beliefs and values inherent in the environments in which expert nurses work.

In Chapter 2 the links between nurses' 'world views' and the knowledge they used and developed was established. Factors, such as management support, shared philosophy and goals, valuing a nursing focus to care, appropriate resources, positive relationships with significant others and authority all contributed to the culture in which nurses worked. Other factors were also influential, such as educational development and reflective ability, and these also have links to the culture.

If we want nurses to be reflective, thinking practitioners, we need to ensure that the culture in which they operate facilitates this process. Resource provision is important in this process and so too is a culture which encourages growth and development. Unfortunately, this was the exception rather than the rule with the expert nurses observed (Conway, 1995). Many areas enforced edicts from above, left staff with inadequate resources and actively discouraged questioning of any kind. The care that developed in some of these areas gave considerable cause for concern.

Openness and challenging

A culture which encourages openness and actively facilitates challenging fosters the development of confident practitioners. Such a culture based on humanistic values enables nurses to feel safe to challenge themselves and others. A lecturer practitioner in such an area described the common philosophy shared by the nurses:

> 'What unites them [the nurses] is that they have a common purpose in their nursing and the philosophy is explicit and is worked with. It really is quite evident that they are working with that common purpose in the way they approach their patient, and that [this] is perceived by patients similarly on questionnaires of their experiences of the ward [which] endorse(s) [this]... One of the things I have enjoyed is facilitating people working through challenges, and they challenge me a fair amount and I've certainly challenged them a fair amount and we have had endless tears, and happy times, and joyful times; I think

that the fact that we have endless niggles is a very healthy sign. It used to worry me initially. I used to say "Oh, ward X does not seem to be happy" and I used to yearn for people saying they were happy...but not recently, I have actually felt happier when I hear of problems rising to the surface and then seeing how they manage those problems.'

The expert nurse here signifies the value she and the other nurses put on the process of challenging. She also highlights an ability to tolerate ambiguity in so much as she perceives niggles and complaints being talked about as a healthy rather than an unhealthy sign. Asked if she was happier when gripes came to the surface because of the sense of honesty, the expert replied:

'I have tended to be very open and approachable, and I have worked very hard at being available and responding very quickly to any tentative half-baked approaches for support or wanting to talk over a problem. Some people bottle out of it; they can't be that honest.'

She also emphasised the importance of mutual intra-professional respect:

'I am fairly supportive of Carl Rogers' view on life. In education I enjoy the open positive regard of students and I see them very much as my equals, and I similarly see my ward staff as my equals.'

Devolution of authority is also important in creating a climate where expertise can develop. Expert nurses such as this used primary nursing as a care delivery method, and decision-making about patient care was devolved to the primary nurse providing care. These experts believed that primary nursing was a significant factor in the development of their expertise:

'Influencing the culture of the place if you like, not only has management devolved from a central position here in nursing but as far as delivery of patient care, it is very much down to individual practising nurses. They have a great deal of autonomy within their own practice. There is obviously a degree of cohesion, sharing of common values if you like. Part of the way we work is that we don't define particularly roles in terms of tasks or activities... we practise primary nursing by that name or another, but basically we are talking about the prospect of a more holistic and individual approach. I do for my patients what my patients need doing, that can encompass anything. If my patients with bowel surgery and bowel prep find themselves with intractable diarrhoea and the loo needs cleaning, then I do it. I would never ever expect not to, or expect to do things that other nurses wouldn't do, or not to do things that other nurses do, ever!'

Professionalism is about being able to care for your own case-load of patients. A holistic nursing focus to care is valued as opposed to attaching significance to any particular task.

Valuing nursing care

Nurses from the group described as Humanistic Existentialist were passionate about nursing. They were politically aware and capable of devising strategies to enable them to develop their practice. They were also very aware of the influence that they had on other nurses.

'I am very credible clinically because I work clinically, and it is quite significant that working clinically at a senior level gives a very clear role model... it clarifies for a number of people the vision of what nursing might be, that's not to say, I am successful all the time, ...there are times when they see very powerful and significant nursing going on, which has been managed and determined by me and that is very important in giving them a clear idea of where they might be going.'

This expert attaches importance to acting as a role model by giving hands-on care. She is aware of the impact she has on other nurses, and she is aware that what she does in terms of care provision is different in that it is 'powerful and significant'. This seems to highlight another difference between the Humanistic expert and other experts, in that Humanistic experts present the process of giving care as being the significant factor rather than a task that is undertaken.

Self-regard

An expert nurse from a medical area identified the importance of valuing yourself before attempting to care for anyone else. She felt that in terms of a general philosophy:

'In order to care for others you have got to care for yourself. I have to have respect and value in my own life, and a value for myself, then I have to have a respect and a care, and maybe an unconditional positive regard for others, but coming from that there has to be an ability, even though it is unconditional, to tell people when they over-step the mark, even patients. "Look, your demands on me today are rather excessive." I will often tell patients, sit down and tell them, what my workload is for the day and explain what is going on in the ward, not giving any confidences away and you know you often get a lot of understanding that way. You make people think outside themselves; sick people are often very introspective, understandably, and so I am not afraid to point out to people when I feel they have overstepped the mark.'

This expert exhibits self-awareness and self-respect in terms of the care she provides. When patients, as she puts it, 'over-step the mark', she is prepared to challenge them by outlining her other duties and responsibilities.

Supervision and support

A supportive type of supervision was in operation in the ward areas in which the Humanistic experts work. One expert nurse who had a dual role as manager-practitioner explained that she worked as an associate nurse a lot and that this was:

> '...in some ways very useful [to] keep my eyes peeled, I take up a lot more in a given time than I think an experienced D grade associate would be able to do. I feed back to the teams, and say I have noticed this, that and the other, "What do you think about that?" I think that is in some ways very useful both for them and for me.'

In terms of providing feedback, the approach this expert nurse outlines sounds friendly and open and is likely to be less threatening than more directive approaches.

Guardians of the culture

Support and encouragement enable nurses to be pro-active in terms of influencing the culture in which they work. Another expert discussed his perception of nurses as guardians of the ward culture:

> 'We are the holders of the culture and we have to keep recreating that culture, we can't actually just let it rest... because it is a very dynamic very complicated situation...'

He raises important issues related to the culture. Because of
the high turnover of medical staff, nurses are a constant
factor at ward level. He highlighted the importance of nurses
re-creating the culture with each new intake of doctors,
presenting this process as essentially dynamic and evolving.

This creation by nurses of the culture seemed to provide
a means whereby expert nurses and their colleagues were
able to establish relationships with the medical staff which
ensured that nursing was recognised and valued:

> 'I suppose from the point of view of the more senior nurses
> on the ward, the approach we take is to keep people
> confronting these situations and to keep confronting them
> ourselves so, rather than just let them rest actually ...we
> need to keep airing these issues; we need to keep
> confronting these issues as they come up ...we are
> guardians of the culture and if we want to have a
> co-operative productive relationship with medical
> colleagues, then that is something we need to keep
> reiterating.'

This expert was motivated to do something positive about
doctor-nurse relationships. First, he felt that nurses needed
to inform the doctor about the way in which they worked at
ward level by discussing their philosophy and the way that
they organise care. Secondly, the expert was realistic about
this process. He conceded that doctors were unlikely to have
time to read information sheets about the nursing position
vis-à-vis care provision on his ward. Thirdly, he and the other
senior staff were prepared to bring about change through a
process of challenging. This type of non-confrontational but
assertive challenging was a hallmark of the Humanistic
Existentialist group (Chapter 2).

Education and relationship to the culture

If we are trying to extend practice and develop expertise in nursing, we need to examine the place of education in this process. Expertise is about much more than simply gaining knowledge of a topic or subject. Indeed, education needs to be a liberating and empowering process (Freire, 1968; 1970; 1973; Jarvis, 1986; Moore, 1989). It appeared that some organisational cultures facilitated this much more than others. Jarvis (1986) describes two types of educational experience — education from above and education of equals:

> *'Education from above is a process whereby the person is moulded to fit into the system, whatever the system may be. Education is, therefore, regarded as essential to the maintenance of the status quo and to the continuity of the system by preparing new recruits to take their place within it without disrupting it. By contrast, the education of equals is a means by which the individual grows and matures, irrespective of the demands of the system'* (Jarvis, 1986: 467).

Education of equals empowers the individual, enabling an active rather than reactive relationship with the social system. Elements of this type of education were operational in the areas in which the humanistic existentialist experts (Chapter 2) worked. Education from above on the other hand, promotes the development of individuals who accept the social system as given and their 'position' within it. This type of educational process was apparent in areas in which traditionalists and some specialists and technologists worked.

Table 6.1: The two educations as curricular models (Jarvis, 1986)

Education from above	Education of equals
Aims:	
Individual should be initiated in the social system and its culture System needs must be met	Individual should be encouraged to achieve his human potential Individual needs should be met
Objectives:	
Specific and behavioural objectives employed	Expressive objectives utilised
Content:	
Selected from the culture group by those delegated by society Initiates individual into publicly accepted knowledge, its forms and structure	Selected from culture of social group(s) by learners often in negotiation with teachers, according to interest and relevance. Problem-based on knowledge, rather than structured
Method:	
Didactic Socratic, when directed towards specific learning outcomes	Facilitative Socratic, when seeking to stimulate learning
Teacher seeks to control learning outcomes. Teacher's role clearly demarcated and regarded as essential to learning	Teacher seeks no control over learning outcomes Teacher's role less clearly demarcated and not regarded as essential to learning
Assessment:	
Public examination Competitive Teacher-set tests Emphasis upon standards	Self-assessment by learner Peer assessment Emphasis on learning

Developing Jarvis's notion of 'education-of-'equals', Moore (1989: 56) offers two conceptions of the ideal nurse.

Table 6.2: Two conceptions of the ideal nurse (Moore, 1989)

Type A Nurse	Type B Nurse
Compliant	Thinking
Obedient	Flexible
Subservient	Problem-solving
Rule-abiding	Autonomous
Policy adhering	Accountable
Procedure following	Self-directed
'Education from above'	'Education of Equals'
Pedagogy	Andragogy
Based on the assumption that the individual is the product of the social system in which he is located.	Based on the assumption that social systems are the product of the individuals who comprise them

When we talk of expertise, it is essential that we identify what we mean. Is an expert compliant, obedient and subservient or is an expert a thinking, flexible, self-directed, autonomous practitioner? Conway argues that it is the latter. Proficiency may be achieved by following procedures and generally being biddable, but developing expertise requires much more than this. Expert practitioners need to be empowered so that they can critically evaluate their practice and the factors which influence it.

> '...one other feature has to be taken into consideration: whether the individual learner is the product of the social system in which s/he is located or whether the system is the product of the persons who comprise it ' (Jarvis, 1986: 466).

The assumption within both Jarvis's and Moore's work is that individuals exposed to 'education-of-equals' are empowered and therefore able to control their social systems rather than being controlled by them.

There are several points of departure between the findings of Conway's study (Conway, 1995) and the suggestions offered by Jarvis and Moore. While the importance of the relationship of the individual to the social system is recognised, findings suggest that the situation is much more complex than utilising an 'education-of-equals' approach.

While education is important, it is not in itself sufficient. Nurses also need authority, support and resources to be able to create and control the social systems within which they work. The assumptions within 'education-of-equals' concurs with the work of Freire (1968; 1970; 1973). Freire focused on dialogue with illiterate Brazilian peasants so that they could relate to their place in creating their culture. Awareness of this relationship empowered them, freeing them to be active in terms of their learning. Nurses in the Humanistic Existentialist group were empowered in a similar way. They were aware of their place in terms of influencing the culture in which they worked and were prepared to take action to support it.

This is an important point but like the chicken and egg, it is difficult to say which comes first. Certainly in her study (Chapter 2), Conway found that humanistic, open, challenging cultures fostered the development of education of equals. Individuals saw themselves as powerful and able to influence events.

In less supportive cultures, individuals saw themselves as powerless in terms of gaining additional resources and in their interactions with others. The following example which occurred during an observation visit to a medical area illustrates this point. The expert was overseeing a number of wards and she visited these in turn. She was asked to describe her thinking as she went round:

Interviewer: *'So what was in your mind as you were going round?'*

Expert: *'Mainly to make sure that they [the staff] were safe really, that they had got adequate staffing levels and that the skill mix was OK. Well, I could see for myself that the skill mix was adequate for each area. They had got sufficient trained nurses to cope and they had got the number that they needed.'*

Interviewer: *'Do you work that out differently every day or do you tend to keep a number in your head..?'*

Expert: *'We have got a number that we are supposed to be working to and the total is five. It used to be six but is now down to five.'*

Interviewer: *'Five?'*

Expert: *'Five total, Five staff. If we can see two trained nurses that's as much as we can expect on a shift you know, which is pretty diabolical, but this morning everywhere we have gone I have seen far more and really that has made me pleased. It has made my day in fact today, because I have seen four and one, and I have got four on here, and there is three on those two [wards] across there. So that has made my day today.'*

Interviewer: *'Are they working with two sometimes?'*

Expert: *'Yes.'*

Interviewer: *'With patients this ill?'*

Expert: *'Yes, yes, it is a very serious situation.'*

This transcript demonstrates the importance that the expert nurse attached to ensuring that at least minimum staffing levels were operational. Also clearly outlined is that the expert nurse recognised that at times staffing levels were 'diabolical', but she did not feel that she could influence this in any way.

From these examples, it can be seen that there are many links between the type of culture in which nurses work and how they grow and develop intellectually and professionally. If we really wish to develop reflective, critically thinking practitioners who are able to deliver high quality care, then cultural influences need serious consideration.

Culture and expert practice

Some might ask how does culture affect nursing practice? Conway has already argued that expertise is about much more than being able to carry out a particular task. When the culture fosters expertise based on a professional model, then very powerful nursing indeed can be realised. The following examples illustrate such nursing in practice. In the first scenario an expert nurse describes an incident where he felt that he really made a difference to a patient care situation.

> 'A lot of things that stick in my mind are like transformative situations. I suppose some of my expertise is in recognising some situations as transformative and illuminating them... For example, quite a few months ago we had a young man on the ward. He had been in a road traffic accident, he was wasted, contracted, he came to us from a rehabilitation unit because he was dehydrated and he had an infection and he became quite physically ill...
>
> Now the hand over that we were given clearly labelled his partner as a trouble-maker. We had comments like "Don't let her interfere" and "She will take control, she will take over", which obviously said to me straight away, "You want control, that's why you feel uncomfortable with her wanting control". There were a couple of us that were intimately involved in the first few days.

What we did was, we just accepted her anxieties, so, rather than trying to challenge her protectiveness, her anxieties, we tried very consciously, the two of us, to accept that that was a very legitimate feeling under the circumstances... she really wanted to be there for him and we converted a sense of being threatened by her wanting to have a degree of control and involvement in his care, to actually using that energy, transforming her emotion into something [in which] we would all be working together... and just recently we were invited to their wedding. We definitely made a significant difference. You could see her relax and start to trust by listening to her...

We were actually saying "We agree with you, you have had a bit of a bad deal. We accept that you want to spend a lot of time with him, we accept that often you will know how to care for him best and certainly you understand and communicate better than we will..." Of course, we are experts in our field and we know about nutrition and we know about hydration and we know about the importance of these things. We know about gastrostomy tubes and we know about pressure sores but none of that is knowledge we can't teach to someone else.

There is no point in being jealous of that professional knowledge. I don't see any of us as being the sorts of people that would hold anything back. We don't want to use knowledge as power... She was quite happy to trust him to our care and she actually had a rest which I though was very good.'

We see here the awareness that this expert nurse has of how support and acceptance can turn a negative situation into a positive one. The expert nurse and his colleague were not prepared to accept the labelling that was given to this patient's fiancée by carers at the home from which he was admitted. The values espoused by this expert were also put into practice in terms of care. These included treating patients as equals and encouraging patients and relatives to make choices and to participate in care. This nurse explained:

'In that particular example, I am not just talking about sharing knowledge, there was also an emotional response. Both of us that were involved in looking after that particular young man and woman in that early situation, were very aware of feeling her distress. Her distress — we very much saw that as a focus for our care.

So our care, which my boss would actually see as something coming out of Buddhism, can also be seen as coming out of Humanism, the idea of actually confronting anxiety, distress, negative fear and trying by one's own good will, one's own unconditional warm regard ...in that situation I can say that that was what I was doing. I did go into that situation where I was accepting, but also I was trying to respond in a human way to the suffering that was going on...

The trouble is the jargon of it, the 'unconditional warm regard' the 'moderated love', those sorts of things, they don't necessarily get across the reality, they don't get across how you feel in those situations and they are poor approximations of what are complex emotions and situations. But I know that I feel things very strongly in certain situations and I know that my colleagues do as well.'

Here the expert nurse recognises that the nursing care he is providing is very sophisticated and complex. It is based on a considered value system and an explicit philosophy of care. The patient's 'condition' alone could have been attended to, but this would have been to deny the importance of the relationship and power distribution between the patient, the fiancée and the nurses. Qualitatively, the patient's treatment was transformed into a positive situation, in which the patient and his fiancée were actively involved and knowledgeable. Care therefore was not just a short-term, here-and-now solution. It was also concerned with the long-term education and development of skills that would be needed for the patient and fiancée to cope in the future.

The nurse was asked what part he felt education played in assisting the development of his expertise. He explained that:

'I would say that my academic work, for want of a better word, does inform my practice and it does so quite strongly, because my academic studies inform my values and it is my values that makes a big difference to how I work.

So the academic... the theoretical and more abstract notions that I have internalised that inform my practice and they do flow out of humanism, they do flow out of a questioning of traditional reductionist knowledge. They do partly flow out of growing spiritual convictions, they certainly flow out of, I hope, quite broad reading...

I don't want to just know about the experience of someone's heart attack. I am interested in knowing what a heart attack does to your myocardium, I am also interested in what it does to your self-image. So it is a broad range... the illnesses are part of the experience, the understanding of the experience comes out of sociology, comes out of psychology and all grey areas in between; it comes out of personal experience... in terms of one's own life and one's own family, going through illness oneself; it also comes out of the extraordinary experience of looking after these people week in, week out.'

This expert demonstrates self-awareness and professional awareness. He presents his practice as a synthesis of knowledge and values.

The following scenarios were described by an expert from a surgical area. They emphasise the centrality of the nurse-patient relationship to the care process. Considerable

integrity is demonstrated in the care given to two patients
who were terminally ill:

'I had two patients recently, who were particularly
poignant because they both asked me to be their primary
nurse. I had promised them both that they could die at
home and that I would do everything I could to facilitate
that happening... One was determined that she wanted
to go home; she was very frightened of dying and we
talked about it up to a point, but we never discussed the
gory details. She knew she was dying. The other one never
really admitted that he was dying... I promised them both
things and I thought about it very carefully... about
whether I had the resources to fulfil those promises and
whether my own personal resources, as well as the
community's resources [would meet the need]...

I did a lot of heart searching about this and it was
extremely painful; it was really very, very difficult... I think
what was very important for me was that the rest of the
team, including the consultant ...we worked together far
more than usually. I think it was brilliant, both for the
consultant and me in terms of credibility, and our working
relationships, but for the rest of the staff to see what we
did and how we did it, was invaluable. They saw how
painful it was and that it was OK to be upset about it.

The woman who went home and died had an upper
gastric carcinoma.. she thought she had beaten it but she
hadn't... she was unable to eat or drink at all, because she
was completely obstructed. Mr A (the surgeon) had known
her for five years. He opened her up and could do nothing
at all, absolutely nothing at all and he was devastated. He
rang me personally, which he has never ever done from
theatre and said please will you come down, I want to talk
about this. I thought it was a bit strange. I knew it was bad
because he would never ever, I have never known him to
do that before...

He said "I want you to keep her comfortable" and I said "What will I do when she asks me, because you know she will ask me" and he said "tell her, you have got to tell her and if I get there first I will tell her". I told her husband what we had found and when she woke the next day I was with her and I told her. I had never had to do that in my professional life before ever, actually be the first person to say, you are going to die because this is what they found. She needed honesty, she needed to be told and she did not need any flapping around or maybe we could do this, or maybe we could do that, and we just said "Fiona, these are the options, it is up to you to choose and we will do whatever you want". She did, she chose and we did what she wanted ...she took her chances and tried to get home...

Getting her home with TPN was the most mammoth problem I have had to deal with for a very long time but we did it, we did it. I will never forget one of the things I said to her before she left was that if she felt at any time that she wanted to withdraw from the TPN and change her mind, that she really had had enough, and she knew that that was feeding her and the tumour and she couldn't keep going, all she had to do was say so, and that was absolutely fine you know. She didn't have to feel that she was committed to it forever and ever until she died, and she did, to my amazement she actually withdrew from it before she died. She was a very brave woman. But I wonder if I had never said it to her if she would have known.

The other case was very different again, because Raymond and his wife refused to believe that he was going to die from this cancer. They were extremely well educated articulate people, it was really quite dumbfounding to them... Eventually his wife Naomi, by this time Raymond was away with the fairies, agreed that he was going... he went downhill very quickly, he died very, very quickly unlike the other lady ...finally his wife accepted that he was going to die, but she did have to tell her children. She had an obligation to inform them of what was going on...

That was very hard for her to accept and I had to, and the associate nurses, I must bring them in, they were all in it, as much involved as me, especially when I am not there, we have to accept that. I helped her to decide to take him home because I knew it was what he wanted although he was past saying so by this stage, he had previously told me that he wanted to go home.'

These two examples demonstrate the degree of commitment this expert nurse had to carrying out her patient's wishes. Because of her sound knowledge base and values, she was able to operate in a sensitive, sophisticated responsive way to both patients' needs.

Not only was she able to organise the support in physical and psychological terms that these patients needed, but she also maintained the trust that both these patients had given to her. It is clear that Fiona (the first patient) was treated as an equal and was fully informed and involved in the decisions about her care. There was no talk of decisions behind closed doors; everything was there for the patient to see and to decide on.

In the second example, even when the patient no longer knew what was happening to him, the expert nurse still kept her word and encouraged the patient's wife to have him home. This signifies a deep moral and ethical commitment. It must surely come from and foster an environment in which patients feel that their wishes are paramount. The care demonstrated in these examples is the antithesis of routinised care. It was clear that the surgeon respected the nurse and treated her as a partner in care, whose advice could be requested. This expert, nurses and the consultant were able to share their feelings through this traumatic experience. The care given was more than a response to a specific situation. The expert carefully thought through what was likely to be involved, before first agreeing to be a primary nurse for these patients. She reflected on her own resources and the support likely to be available in the community. Only then had she decided that she would agree to the patients' requests. Consideration and thoughtfulness permeate these examples and demonstrate the powerful nature of the nursing commitment shown by this expert nurse. The culture this nurse worked in enabled expertise of this type to develop and flourish.

Conclusion

If we wish to develop expert nursing such as in these examples, we need to acknowledge the influence of culture on practitioners. The totality of nurses' 'world views' needs attention. Support from management is essential. Nurses need to be able to direct their energy towards pro-active high quality care, rather than feeling powerless and undervalued by managers who have separate agendas. While educational input is essential to underpin any advancement, this needs to be not only of subject matter knowledge but also empowering in nature. Nurses who truly operate from a nursing focus to care do much more than simply carry out a number of tasks. Such care is to be fostered, rather than reducing such richness to a number of tasks.

References

Conway JE (1995) *Expert Nursing Knowledge as an Evolutionary Process*. Unpublished PhD Thesis. University of Warwick, Coventry

Freire P (1968) *Pedagogy of the Oppressed*. Herder and Herder, New York

Freire P (1970) *Cultural Action for Freedom*. Penguin Books, Middlesex

Freire P (1973) *Education for Critical Consciousness*. Sheed and
Ward, London

Jarvis P (1986) Janforum: Nurse education and adult education:
a question of the person. *J Adv Nurs* **11**: 465–9

Moore DJ (1989) Educating Adults. In: Bradshaw PL ed.
Teaching and Assessing in Clinical Practice. Prentice Hall,
London: 38–63

Chapter 7

What now? Some final considerations

What is the nurse's role to be in the future? Is it to be mini-doctor, maxi-nurse, Technologist, Traditionalist, Specialist, Humanistic Existentialist? It seems that 'you pays your money and you take your choice'. The road ahead for nursing is about choice, some of which may be painful. But who are the people making the choices for nursing? What are their concerns? As one expert put it:

> 'As nurses go higher up in management, they tell you that their concern is the budget.'

While it may well be a fact of life that we all have to work within finite budgets, we need to ensure that the vision of what nursing can be is not subsumed by budgetary concerns. Nursing is facing a crisis of identity. It is pulled in one direction by service needs yet striving at the same time to achieve both academic and professional recognition. Reconciling such conflicts will be no mean task.

We need to debate the influence of such tensions on nursing. This is partly the reason for writing this book. If the 'selective blindness of the oppressed' shown by some experts in this work is to be overcome, nurses need to be empowered so that they can cope with looking searchingly at themselves and their practice. Empowerment is much more than a popular cliché of the moment. It is about support, role models and feeling valued. It is about striving for professional maturity.

Indeed, the debate goes beyond this. It is about articulating the 'worth' of professional practice in non-reductionist terms. Competency approaches for evaluating nursing go some way only towards identifying the specialness of nursing. Nursing is much more than a number of tasks. The scenarios in this work capture some of this specialness. They demonstrate the importance of intangibles such as integrity and humanism. They expose the reality of what expert nurses using a professional base to practice can do.

To be an advocate for someone else, you first have to be able to stand up for yourself. To influence events, you need a positive sense of your own self-worth. Sound knowledge and passion in terms of nursing care have been captured in many of these scenarios. I hope that they will provide a sense of possibility for those who feel powerless and oppressed within their working culture. Change is possible.

Index